Time to Talk
Parents' Accounts of Children's
Speech Difficulties

Time to Talk

Parents' Accounts of Children's Speech Difficulties

MARGARET GLOGOWSKA PhD, MRCSLT

Frenchay Hospital, Bristol

Consulting Editor in
Developmental Speech and Language Therapy
JANET LEES
Department of Human Communication Science
University of Sheffield

W
WHURR PUBLISHERS
LONDON AND PHILADELPHIA

© 2002 Whurr Publishers Ltd
First published 2002
by Whurr Publishers Ltd
19b Compton Terrace
London N1 2UN England and
325 Chestnut Street, Philadelphia PA 19106 USA

British Library Cataloguing in Publication Data

A catalogue record for this book
is available from the British Library.

ISBN 1 86156 305 1

Printed and bound in the UK by Athenaeum Press Ltd,
Gateshead, Tyne & Wear.

Contents

Preface

This book is about the experience of having a child who has early difficulties with learning to talk. It is based on the accounts of the parents of 20 children who took part in a wider research project. This project ran between 1995 and 1999 in the Speech and Language Therapy Research Unit, Frenchay Hospital, Bristol. It was funded by the Research and Development Directorate of the South West NHS Executive. At the end of their involvement in the project, the parents agreed to take part in in-depth interviews where they talked about their experience of early speech and language delays and how these affected their child and their family. They also spoke about the help they sought for the difficulties, the progress made by the child in their speech and language development and their hopes for their child's future progress.

During the time in which the interviews took place, it became clear that the parents were grappling with a number of issues including:

- trying to make sense of the early difficulties experienced by their children
- wanting to know more about the difficulties but not knowing where to look
- coping with the emotional issues of having a child experiencing speech and language difficulties
- knowing few other parents with children experiencing similar problems, to whom they could talk about what was happening
- being concerned about the referral of their child to speech and language therapy for the difficulties.

The idea for this book sprang from the stories of these parents. It was clear that early speech and language delays were often poorly understood by the parents, leading to feelings of isolation and fear when they encountered difficulties in their child's development of speech and language. The interviews with the parents suggested that they wanted more information about the difficulties and what attendance at speech and language therapy might entail. The parents also expressed a range of feelings at the beginning of their involvement in speech and language therapy and their need of emotional support and reassurance at this time.

At the time of the interviews publications were available which gave parents information about the course of normal development and advice about ways in which parents could help when difficulties arose. However, there was little information the parents could draw on which dealt specifically with early speech and language difficulties and beginning speech and language therapy for children. One area in which there was no information for parents, before or after referral to speech and language therapy, was that of the opinions and perceptions of other parents whose children had been referred to speech and language therapy for a speech and language problem in their pre-school years. This book, therefore, is the first account of early speech and language difficulties written almost entirely from the perspective of parents. It seems appropriate that an account of the experiences of parents, as told by parents, should be available so that parents and others can benefit from it. It is widely accepted that a gap exists between research carried out in health services and the information it generates becoming available to patients and carers. There is huge variability in the effort which is put into making research findings accessible to people who are not professionals. This book is part of an attempt to ensure that the findings of this research did not just gather dust on library shelves or only be quoted by other researchers.

The book is written to convey the experiences of the parents in coming to terms with their children's speech and language difficulties and seeking help for them. In Chapter 1, the parents describe the features of their children's speech and language which first raised their concerns and their own ideas about what may have caused the difficulties. Chapter 2 is an account of the parents' attempts to get professional help for their children and their feelings about the referral of their children to speech and language therapy, while the third chapter deals with the first visit to speech and language therapy. Chapters 4 and 5 document the views of parents about the therapy options they experienced and their perceptions on the process of therapy. Chapter 6 considers the views the parents expressed on the research itself and the meaning their participation in the project held for them. In Chapter 7, the parents describe their children's progress and talk about the hopes they have for their children's further development. Chapter 8 takes an overview of all the parents' accounts and discusses the common themes running through them. It also goes on to explore advice and suggestions made by the parents both for other parents experiencing a similar situation and for professionals. A detailed account of how the study was carried out is given in the Appendix.

Readers interested in exploring some issues in more depth will find a list of relevant texts in the Further Reading section. A list of useful addresses is given at the end of the book.

In order to tap into the diversity of parents' experiences, a range of parents from differing backgrounds and circumstances was selected for interview. However, in the wider project, children from homes where English was not the only language were not included, as there is evidence that children's learning of two or more languages is different from children's learning of a single language. Including bilingual children in research into early delays may complicate an already quite complex picture. For that reason, it was not possible to interview parents from ethnic minority backgrounds. It is entirely possible that parents from ethnic minorities could have differing expectations and experiences of health care services, cultural assumptions and social support networks. For this reason, the perceptions of these parents about early speech and language difficulties and speech and language therapy could vary enormously from those of the parents who were interviewed. It would be wrong, however, to assume that this is the case. This book is not able to contribute to our knowledge of this particular topic but the experiences of parents from ethnic minorities clearly demand much more research.

In the past, books about speech and language difficulties have often been written from professional, clinical, medical and academic perspectives. This book breaks with tradition in this respect as it presents the difficulties from the points of view of those who have lived with them on a day-to-day basis. Therefore, in each chapter of the book, the emphasis is on showing what the parents believed and felt about the difficulties and the speech and language therapy service they received, as far as possible in the words they used themselves. In a number of the chapters, however, the parents' accounts are supplemented with other information based, in the main, on research findings. The purpose of this approach is to acknowledge the importance of the views of parents but also to present their views within the wider context to which they belong. It is my hope that in telling the stories of parents alongside the giving of factual information, both can be seen as equally valid perspectives on early speech and language delays.

The book has been written, first and foremost, with parents in mind. I hope that parents of children with speech and language delays will find it helpful, not only as a source of information about the difficulties themselves and what can be done to help them but also as a source of support, as they cope with the everyday difficulties and frustrations of living with speech and language difficulties. Parents' need for reliable and useful information has never been greater, as within the National Health Service of today, there is an increasing emphasis on shared clinical decision-making. Clients and their carers are becoming increasingly involved in the delivery of health care. However, such a process relies heavily on clients and carers having the information necessary to answer their questions and help them make choices about what should happen in their health care. Because its primary audience is parents, the layout of the book has been designed to be as straightforward as possible. The language of the book is accessible to those without any knowledge of speech and language difficulties. To keep the text as simple and uncluttered as possible, referencing is not used.

As well as being a resource for parents, it is hoped that this book will be of interest to all professionals who come into contact with pre-school children and who may be unaware of the impact of the difficulties and referral to speech and language therapy on the parents of the children affected. Those working within charitable organizations offering support to children with speech and language difficulties and their parents may find that the book raises issues affecting their work. Finally, I hope that the book will be thought-provoking for speech and language therapists and their managers, as I feel it should support them in the planning and delivery of services which are responsive to the needs of children, their parents and their wider family.

At this point, I would like to acknowledge all those who made this book possible. While the speech and language therapy project itself was funded by the Research and Development Directorate of the South West NHS Executive, the writing of this book has been supported entirely by the Underwood Trust. I owe a debt of thanks to the other members of the team working on this project – Dr Sue Roulstone, Dr Tim Peters and Professor Pam Enderby. They have been closely involved in the planning and writing of this book and have made many useful suggestions. I am also extremely grateful to Dr Rona Campbell, who was instrumental in shaping the design of the project and ensuring that the research was conducted in a systematic and rigorous way. At every stage, I have relied on her understanding of the investigation, her guidance and her questioning of the interpretation of the material collected from the parents. I am grateful to Janet Lees for her constructive comments and supportive editing of the book. At the Speech and Language Therapy Research Unit, Shirley Cotton has been a constant source of support and practical help. I would also like to acknowledge the personal help I have received from Henryk and Anna Glogowscy.

Last but certainly not least, I would like to express my sincere thanks to the parents whose accounts I have had the privilege of hearing. It is my hope that their willingness to share their experiences will be translated by this book into a source of support for other parents.

Margaret Glogowska
September 2001

CHAPTER 1

Speech and language delays – what are they like and why do they happen?

BOX 1.1 SPEECH AND LANGUAGE DELAYS: SOME FACTS

Speech and language delays can affect young children's understanding of spoken language, their use of single words and putting together of words to communicate and their ability to produce speech which others are able to understand.

Sometimes speech and language delays can be linked to difficulties with hearing, general learning problems, cerebral palsy and emotional disturbances. However, speech and language delays can also occur in children who have no other problems.

Speech and language delays are common. About a fifth of parents are worried about their children's speech and language development at any one time.

About six per cent of all children are experiencing some form of difficulties with speech or language.

Boys are three to four times more likely than girls to experience speech and language delays.

She wasn't speaking, she had no babble, she didn't have any form of communication at all . . . she was a very silent child which was why we went through hearing tests. We felt that she may have a real hearing problem but she just wasn't communicating and intermingling at all with any child. She wouldn't sort of interact in any way, shape or form, she wouldn't be able to show how she felt but she was very frustrated. **Emma**

I think it was her, I think it was 18 months or a bit older than that . . . the woman there [*the health visitor*] sort of gave her bricks and said 'Put the red brick on the blue brick' and . . . and she wasn't really responding and she showed her things in a book . . . she didn't really respond very well to that. **Monica**

I think it was his 18 month visit at home. You know, she [*the health visitor*] did all the normal checks and asked all the normal questions and everything was fine except for she said that he should be saying a fair number of words and he wasn't. **Caroline**

He started speaking very late . . . by sort of 18 months, two years he was just saying the . . . odd word . . . very, very simple words . . . like 'Mum', 'Dad', not a lot and as he began to say more, by the time he got to just under three . . . everything he said never had beginnings on it and nobody could understand. **Sally**

He failed most of his hearing tests when he was small and . . . and a lot of his sounds weren't that clear and I was a little bit concerned about him because . . . he wasn't making himself understood properly and he was getting quite frustrated about it. **Patricia**

He had one of his check-ups with the health visitor and she felt his speech wasn't . . . how it should be and she also sent him for a hearing test as well and they checked his hearing and his hearing was fine but . . . they felt that he needed to be observed for his speech. **Bernadette**

Emma, Monica, Caroline, Sally, Patricia and Bernadette are talking about their children who had difficulties early on with their speech and language development. Emma describes how her two-and-a-half-year-old daughter was unable to communicate and interact with people at all. Monica's two-year-old daughter found it very difficult to understand sentences and questions she was asked. Caroline and her health visitor became concerned when her two-year-old son was only using a few, simple words to communicate. After a late start in talking, Sally's three-year-old boy could not be understood by his family and friends. Patricia's three and a half year old son had repeatedly failed hearing tests and also experienced problems in making himself understood. At three-and-a-half, Bernadette's little boy's speech sounds were not always clear and he was referred to speech and language therapy. For many parents, their children's first words are an eagerly awaited event and learning to talk an enjoyable, exciting process to observe and be involved in. However, as these parents' accounts show, children can meet difficulties when they are learning to talk which affect them and their families. Such problems can range from children not interacting with others, not understanding what is said to them, using few words to communicate with others to not being easily understood by those around them.

Becoming aware of early speech and language difficulties

The extracts from interviews with Emma, Monica, Caroline, Sally, Patricia and Bernadette reveal the patterns in their children's talking which made them aware initially that their child was experiencing problems. When quotations are used in this book, hesitations which occur in the parents' speech are indicated by dots (. . .). Occasionally, dots are also used to indicate where a sentence or a block of speech has been left out because it is not relevant to the point the parent is making.

For the slightly younger children (aged two to two-and-a-half years), parents noticed difficulties with *language* – the children were having trouble understanding or using words to communicate. For the older children (aged three years and on), parents were aware of their children's difficulties with *speech* – the children were finding it difficult to make themselves understood. Sometimes parents considered both speech and language development together. Sally, describing her son's speech difficulties, mentioned that his language development had also been slow:

> He started speaking very late . . . by sort of 18 months, two years he was just saying the . . . odd word . . . very, very simple words . . . like 'Mum', 'Dad', not a lot.

Some parents were aware of even earlier patterns in their children's development. Emma commented on how her daughter had not babbled as a baby:

> She wasn't speaking, she had no babble . . . she was a very silent child.

There were sometimes particular circumstances which made their children's difficulties stand out. For Sally, it was the frustration shown by her little boy when he could not make himself understood by members of the family:

> He was getting very cross with everybody, very frustrated and it was just getting worse and worse and worse.

Fiona's son had experienced bouts of *otitis media* early on in his life. Also known as glue ear, this is a condition produced by an infection in the middle ear, which can result in hearing loss. While improvements had come about in his hearing, his talking continued to lag behind:

> I felt that there had been some improvement in his hearing so I was thinking maybe there was something else and this was the time to start helping his speech.

Hearing difficulties appeared to be a common problem among these children and parents often mentioned that their child's hearing was being investigated at the same time that concerns about speech and language arose. For some parents, other aspects of their child's development and medical conditions, as well as speech and language, had given cause for concern. These children were usually being seen by hospital consultants and other professionals:

> He was going through quite a bit 'cos he was going for regular check-ups at the Children's Hospital . . . he was having a lot of problems with his asthma and he was on various medication. **Bernadette**

> Not only did we have problems with her speech we have problems with her social skills as well and development which she's under a paediatrician so in general at that particular time was a very bad time for us. **Emma**

In other respects, however, the children were often felt to be developing well:

> He was quiet . . . but you know really good with other things, playing, jigsaws and colouring, all those sort of things but just quiet. **Caroline**

> I mean he was developing in every other area well . . . he was mixing with other children, you know, doing anything a normal child would do. **Linda**

For some of the parents, the fact that the child was doing well in other aspects of development made the speech and language delay all the more puzzling. However, one mother pointed out that her son's abilities in other areas of development reassured her that he was learning skills in his own way and that his speech and language development were, therefore, no cause for concern:

> He was just doing it all so differently [*from his sister*]. I mean his coordination was so good and . . . I was always being amazed, what he could do, what he could climb. **Sandra**

'You try not to but you can't help it': comparing the child with others

All the parents described how comparing the child with others had made them aware that their child was experiencing difficulties with learning to talk. The parents usually compared the child with brothers and sisters or other children in the family. Occasionally when the child did not have brothers or sisters the child was compared with children outside the family at playgroups and other pre-school settings:

> Well, the problem was, we were comparing him with my daughter who was very, very quick. **Carol**

> When you compare with other children he just wasn't saying anything. **Linda**

> I compared her to her friends and she was very, very far behind. **Hayley**

A number of parents felt that it was a natural thing to make comparisons between children but still felt that it was something that they should not do, because children develop in their own unique way. However, as this father's statement shows, parents found it hard to avoid making comparisons especially when the differences between the children were very obvious:

> You try not to but you can't help but to, can you, 'cos I mean everybody says they all walk at different stages and they all talk at different stages . . . but you try not to compare them but yeah, you find yourself not, well you can't help it can you, because, especially if yours is the only one that's not really communicating and everybody else's is communicating. **Gary**

For all the parents, the act of comparing their child with others increased their concern about their child's difficulties.

What causes early speech and language difficulties?

When describing how they became aware of their child's speech and language difficulties, the parents also talked about possible causes of the difficulties. They expressed a range of ideas about what might have brought about the problems their children were experiencing. These are shown in Box 1.2.

BOX 1.2 IDEAS ABOUT THE CAUSES OF EARLY SPEECH AND LANGUAGE DIFFICULTIES DESCRIBED BY THE PARENTS

Medical reasons.

Parents' actions.

Family background.

The children themselves.

Medical reasons

Where the children had experienced medical problems, their parents often made the connection between them and their child's speech and language difficulties. A number of parents related their child's talking difficulties to the hearing problems. Other medical causes mentioned by the parents were problems with tonsils and adenoids which required surgery, premature birth, difficulties with the birth resulting in slow development and convulsions or fits. The parents also questioned the effects of physical features in their children such as the activity of the tongue or the size of the mouth, the throat and vocal cords.

Actions of the parents

The parents were convinced that their own actions had a part to play in shaping their child's speech and language development. A few parents thought that they might not have spent enough time in stimulating their child's language:

> I just thought perhaps we weren't spending time sitting down and talking as much as we could have. **Carol**

and that acceptance of the child's non-verbal communication, such as pointing, meant that there was no need for the child to use language to communicate:

> So perhaps I never did encourage him like I should have done . . . I could understand what he was trying to tell me, you know, just a couple of grunts and a couple of points or just the way he shrieked at me. **Sandra**

One mother mentioned that her son had not been allowed to speak incorrectly during the time he was developing language which she felt could lead to problems:

> It's not really the case that he sort of learned a gobbledygook language that we all let him get away with and he doesn't have to speak properly. **Caroline**

Another parent felt that demands on her child's communication when he started playgroup might have led to his difficulties:

> I would have said the only problems . . . in the way he was, was probably at playgroup, they said he was really, really quiet. **Amy**

Sometimes the parents questioned how they had raised their children and wondered whether they had given them the chance to spend enough time mixing with children of their own age or whether going to a childminder meant that the child had missed out on being with other children developing language. A few parents also talked about their toddlers' use of dummies and bottles:

> I mean his actual problem was isolated to those sounds and I think the lady had some theories about what would have caused it . . . and it might have been the dummy at night. **Ross**

The parents accepted that using dummies and bottles might not be ideal for children's development of speech but felt that they were necessary items and that limited use was unlikely to have been the only cause of the difficulties.

Some parents also called into question their own lifestyle and personality in trying to make sense of the difficulties their child was experiencing:

> We're all quite a talkative bunch, you know, we're out and about and he goes to the crèches every morning and mixes with other people and other children. **Caroline**

They saw important connections between the child's problem and family stresses that had taken place such as redundancy and moving home. They also linked the difficulties to the way in which television had become a big feature of their child's everyday life. As one mother reported:

> I'm a bit of a stickler about television. I don't like television being on. **Fiona**

Some parents, however, were convinced that only extreme actions, such as not speaking to children at all or not involving them in day-to-day household activities, could cause problems.

Family background

A family history of difficulties was also mentioned by some parents. Either they had experienced problems with talking themselves or their other children had. Very few parents assumed that because these difficulties had been present in the family it was inevitable that other children would experience them. The parents did feel, however, that family background could influence their children's talking in other ways. The parents often believed that the presence, or absence, of brothers and sisters could sometimes be a disadvantage. Where the child had no siblings, parents felt that lack of another child to copy could lead to difficulties:

I thought maybe it was that he had no sibling to . . . to learn from. **Andrea**

Where the child was first in the family, the lack of someone to follow was thought to be negative but the presence of a 'quicker' younger sibling could also disrupt language learning in the elder child:

I do often think maybe it was because she chatted so well and took over everything. **Amy**

Where the child was lower down in the birth order, such as second or third, it was assumed that the child would almost definitely be a slower language learner, because the child was competing with brothers and sisters to be heard:

He was fighting for his own bit of space in a way, I suppose to get the proper attention that he needed to make himself understood. **Patricia**

or because the child's brothers and sisters were prepared to do the talking for him:

If he couldn't get it across he'd give up . . . somebody else would work it out. She'd [*child's sister*] do it for him anyway. **Bernadette**

or because the child was recognizing that his own communication was inferior to that of his older brothers and sisters:

Maybe it was because we had another two children . . . and maybe he thought I don't sound like that, I won't bother. **Ross**

The children themselves

The parents who were interviewed questioned whether their child's social development played a part in the difficulties. Instead of concentrating on learning language, the child was choosing to focus on non-language based activities:

He wasn't so much vocal but he would play. He was very into physical play. **Sandra**

and not being inclined to listen and learn:

His personality, running around, busy, busy, busy, you know, he wouldn't want you to waffle on to him about things. **Sandra**

The parents viewed their children as taking an active part in their own development and not being taught skills passively. Some parents saw their child's delay in speech and language as a decision made by the child to develop in this area at his own speed. The child's personality and emotional characteristics were also thought by parents to play an important part in language learning. Where the child was thought to be lazy or stubborn, lacking in confidence or not wanting to look stupid, language development could be a slower process. Parents did appear to take it for granted that boys were unlikely to learn to talk as quickly and as well as girls.

The parents' feelings about early speech and language difficulties

Coming from different places, backgrounds and families, the parents interviewed described their child's difficulties in different ways and had different ideas about what might have caused them. But in spite of these differences, there were similarities in the way they felt about their child's difficulties, as Box 1.3 shows.

Box 1.3 Feelings expressed by the parents about their children's early speech and language delays

Puzzled.

Struggling to understand why the difficulties have happened.

Uncertain about possible causes of the difficulties.

Guilty because they might be at fault.

For many children who experience speech and language delays, there is no obvious 'cause' of their difficulties, although other difficulties such as hearing loss might have occurred. Where this was the case, the parents often appeared to be extremely puzzled about their child's difficulty and questioned why the difficulties were present:

He started talking late but why I don't know. **Sally**

I mean he was developing in every other area well, so no, can't see why there was, should be any other reason really. **Linda**

I don't really know why she's been the one. **Selina**

When considering the cause of their children's difficulties, most parents believed that single factors acting alone were probably not enough to lead to the difficulties. They remained uncertain, however, about what other things might have contributed. This seemed to make them more likely to question themselves. They wondered whether or not they could be to blame for the difficulties. They were aware of things they had done or had failed to do and felt a great deal of responsibility, as Emma's remark shows:

> I suppose you always sort of question yourself and question your family and have you done it right.

The parents sometimes felt led to believe by professionals that they had been the cause of the child's problems. Caroline related how she felt her actions were being criticized and blamed for her son's difficulties:

> When he was two, he still drank from a bottle in the morning and when he went to bed but he had his cup during the day and it was, 'Oh no, no, no, get rid of that bottle, he doesn't want that bottle, that won't be helping him with his speech.'

Making sense of the difficulties

Because children so often learn to talk without experiencing any difficulties, parents can take it for granted that language development will come about. The majority of the parents who took part in this project had other children who learned language easily. When they then went on to have a child who experienced problems with speech and language, they found it difficult to understand and accept. The parents sought ways of explaining how the difficulties could have happened. They made connections between the talking difficulties and medical problems experienced by the child.

The parents questioned what effects their own actions might have had on their child. They were anxious, also, about the possible effects of family size and order of birth of their child. As part of coming to terms with the difficulties, parents tried hard to make sense of what was going on in their child's lives and very often ended up blaming themselves for what was happening. Occasionally, the parents did realize that they could not be at fault. As Carol explains, when she looked at the situation more objectively, she knew that she had not treated her little boy any differently from his elder sister and yet the problems had still occurred:

I did feel very guilty at first, 'cos perhaps I should've done more for him . . . we've done exactly the same with him as what we done with his sister really but you do go through those emotions.

What is known about early speech and language delays

Professionals, just like parents, do not have all the answers about speech and language delays and why they come about. However, the research which has been carried out into the delays up until now suggests that:

- While hearing problems may be important in the course of individual children's speech and language difficulties, they do not explain the majority of speech and language delays.
- Children's speech and language delays have not been strongly linked with difficulties occurring during their birth.
- The language environment the child is growing up in is rarely the only cause of the difficulties. While parents can influence their child's development of speech and language, the child's delay may also affect the language the parent uses with the child.
- With regard to family size and birth order, large families may reduce the opportunity for children to communicate with adults. It is unlikely, however, that such factors could be solely to blame for the difficulties.

Bilingual children and early speech and language delays

The research project, of which the interviews with the parents formed part, only investigated speech and language delays in children learning one language. No children from homes where a language other than English was spoken were included in the project. This means that no parents from ethnic minority backgrounds could be included in the interviews. It is not possible to predict in which ways the views of such parents might be similar to, or vary from, those presented in this book. More research is necessary to find out what families from ethnic minorities think about speech and language delays and the speech and language therapy services that are available to them. However, what is known about bilingualism and early speech and language delays is summarized in Box 1.4.

Box 1.4 Bilingualism and early speech and language delays: what is known

Children who grow up in homes where more than one language is spoken are not at greater risk of experiencing speech and language delays.

Children who are being raised bilingually, however, may have a preferred language which they use more easily than the other. This may depend on the need and opportunities the child has to use each language.

If a bilingual child is referred to speech and language therapy, the speech and language therapist will be trying to discover whether the child is having a problem with learning language generally or just learning a specific language. Therefore, in assessing whether a child growing up in a bilingual environment is experiencing a delay, the child's ability in all languages should be taken into account. One language may be developing more quickly than another.

Factors making the parents decide to seek help

When they first became aware that their children might be finding talking difficult, some parents discussed the child with their health visitor and were happy to monitor the child's progress for a few months themselves. The parents hoped that during this period of time their child would improve to the point where they no longer had a problem. When the problems did not lessen, a number of factors made the parents decide to seek help. These are listed in Box 1.5.

Box 1.5 The parents' reasons for seeking help

The child is saying very little or is very difficult to understand.

The child is becoming upset or frustrated.

The child seems to be lagging behind his or her friends in talking.

The child is also experiencing hearing difficulties.

When their children were still saying very little or were still very difficult to understand, the parents were very concerned:

I suppose yeah, it was the complete lack of any, of very very limited speech, that was the main, yeah the main incentive for seeking help really. **Isabel**

The effects the difficulties were having on the children's lives were also important to the parents at this point, particularly where the children were becoming frustrated or upset themselves:

Well, I felt that he needed help because he was just getting crosser and crosser . . . and he was suffering himself from it, because he was getting so cross with his little friends at playgroup . . . 'cos they couldn't understand him, you know, something needed to be done, to help him out of the situation that he was in. **Sally**

The parents were now specifically judging how the child seemed in comparison with other children of the same age. When they felt their child was falling behind by quite a long way, the parents wanted to act:

She was very, very far behind. So I just pushed it even more. **Hayley**

The parents were also considering how other difficulties, such as hearing loss, might be interfering with speech and language development and whether they should be doing something about the speech and language difficulties:

We didn't really know whether it was glue ear or not, and if it wasn't then I wanted to do something, you know, get moving. **Fiona**

For these reasons, the parents really felt that help was necessary. The next chapter will explore what the parents went on to do about the difficulties and how their children came to be referred to speech and language therapy services.

Summary of the chapter
- Children can experience problems with learning to talk which may affect their interaction with others, their understanding, how they put words together and how easy to understand they are.
- The parents interviewed in this study had become aware of their child's difficulties by the time the child was two to three years old.
- The parents often compared the progress of the child with his/her brothers and sisters or other children they knew.
- Very often, the parents expressed their own ideas about possible causes of their child's difficulties.

- Research has shown that speech and language delays are linked with some other developmental problems. Bilingual children are not more likely to be delayed in their speech and language development.
- Many of the parents felt they might be to blame for their child's difficulties but this is unlikely to be the case.
- The parents sometimes monitored their child's progress in speech and language with their health visitor.
- If improvement did not come about within a few months, the parents went on to seek referral to speech and language therapy.

CHAPTER 2

Being referred to speech and language therapy

The parents who took part in the interviews seemed to realize gradually that their child's speech and language development was not proceeding as it should. They were not always sure whether their child really did have a problem and their uncertainty went on for some time. Learning to talk is a complex process involving many different skills. There are enormous variations in children's speech and language abilities during the pre-school period, all of which would be considered entirely normal. This makes it even harder to pick out real difficulties from problems which will right themselves in time or normal development which is just proceeding more slowly. For the first-time parents in particular, identifying whether a problem existed was even more difficult, when they had no other child of their own with whom they could make comparisons. The vast majority of the parents, however, did get to the point where they felt that the difficulties were not getting better and wanted to find out what could be done for their children. This chapter will consider how the children were referred to speech and language therapy and how their parents felt about the referral.

Talking to the health visitor

Nearly all the parents who took part in the interviews mentioned that they had talked to their health visitor about their children's speech and language difficulties. A number of parents mentioned that, when they were first becoming aware that their child was experiencing difficulties with talking, with the guidance of their health visitor they kept a close eye on their children's speech and language development for a period of a few months. During this time they were hoping that the child would start saying more words, put more words together or become clearer:

> I think it was, well it was the health visitor as well and me. We just noticed . . . he
> just wasn't talking and what he was saying wasn't clear . . . but she [*the health*

visitor] said they can develop all of a sudden. Then I think I phoned her after about three months. **Linda**

I mean the health visitor was helpful but initially she wasn't too concerned and then I rang her again and expressed more concern. **Isabel**

Ways in which referral to speech and language therapy came about

The parents described a number of ways in which referral of their child to speech and language therapy went ahead, as shown in Box 2.1. Most referrals of young children to speech and language therapy come about in one of these ways.

BOX 2.1 HOW REFERRAL TO SPEECH AND LANGUAGE THERAPY CAME ABOUT

By talking with the health visitor at a routine developmental check.

By contacting the health visitor specially.

Through a visit to the family's GP.

By the parents directly referring the child themselves.

When the expected changes did not happen, these parents reported going back to the health visitor. Some parents were able to discuss their child's problems at the routine developmental checks which take place at around 18 months and three-and-a-half-years. Other parents specially contacted their health visitor because of their concerns about their child's speech and language development. Many of the parents had become sure that a problem did exist and involving the health visitor confirmed this. The health visitor then recommended referring the child to speech and language therapy, as these parents' accounts show:

I'd noticed that he . . . wasn't so clear, his speaking wasn't clear and then at his three year check the health visitor noticed as well 'cos she said to me . . . 'He's not clear' and I said 'Yeah' so she referred him. **Amy**

I went to see the health visitor and asked, I didn't think he was . . . speaking as well as he should do . . . and she said 'Yeah I think he should be referred'. **Andrea**

I went to the . . . you know they have the check-up every so often . . . and I just didn't think he was talking as much as he should be and I mentioned it when I went there and they said 'Yeah, right' and 'We'll refer him to speech therapy'. **Kate**

Not all parents approached their health visitor to discuss their child's difficulties and to seek help. One parent visited her GP so that her daughter could be referred to speech and language therapy. Another mother who herself worked in child health referred her son to the speech and language therapist.

Identifying early speech and language delays

In the interviews, the parents described their increasing awareness of their child's speech and language difficulties. Yet they often lacked confidence in their judgement that something really was wrong, even when they had had previous experience of early speech and language difficulties. They went on to describe how they approached child health professionals to find out whether something needed to be done to help their child. However, it is not just parents who may feel unsure about the presence of early speech and language difficulties in their children. Within speech and language therapy, there is no generally agreed upon definition of what constitutes speech and language delay. Similarly, there is no single process which has been shown to identify best these types of delay. Because of this, there is a debate in speech and language therapy over the extent to which parents should be involved in the screening of children for early speech and language delays and how their role should fit in with that of professionals. Some researchers have recommended an increase in the involvement of parents in identifying problems, as parents are in the best position to observe how their child communicates in everyday life and the impact of any difficulties. There is also research which suggests that parents' reports can be as accurate in identifying difficulties as the screening tests which are currently being used for this purpose.

The parents' feelings about referral

The parents had heard a number of arguments about the timing of referral to speech and language therapy and whether or not children needed to be referred when they were very young, as these statements reveal:

> Some people say 'Oh, they, you know, children always learn to speak. He'll do it, they just rush in', you know. Other people were like, 'No, no, it would be good, it might sort of help him', things like that. So I just sort of thought it would, if it helps the situation then it's good. **Caroline**

> Generally, it was, you know, mums worry about too many things . . . it'll sort itself out . . . which is fine if it does . . . we don't want to wait and find out six months, a year later that it wasn't going to sort itself out and we really have got big problems with the child as a result. **Fiona**

Sometimes the parents did feel frustrated by the advice they were given by friends and family members who wanted to reassure them that the difficulties would sort themselves out. As this mother's comments show, she felt that others around her were not taking note of the problem when they should have done so:

> Everybody's got an opinion about children's speech and especially like relatives and friends and everybody used to say, 'Don't worry, she'll be fine' . . . I mean it could be very dismissive really that people didn't tend to take this too seriously, you know, when you expressed your concerns. **Isabel**

'Earlier rather than later': positive feelings about referral

However, the vast majority of parents made the decision to come forward for referral to speech and language therapy when their children were toddlers and believed that sooner is better than later. Carol felt that it was essential to deal with any problems early on and that parents should not hesitate in seeking help:

> There are children at my daughter's school now in her class they're still having speech problems . . . 'cos their parents never bothered to get it [*try to deal with the problem*] early.

While the parents, on the whole, wanted referral to speech and language therapy to go ahead, they experienced a range of feelings and emotions about the process. For the most part, the parents said they felt pleased and relieved about referral:

> Well it was what I wanted so I was very happy. **Fiona**

> I mean I was glad it was being dealt with, straightaway, yeah. **Amy**

Referral to speech and language therapy was seen by many of the parents as reassuring. They felt positive that if the child did have real difficulties these could be identified and dealt with. The parents also felt that the earlier a problem was recognized the better:

> I was quite pleased 'cos I thought, well, at least it means that someone's taking notice that there is a problem. **Selina**

> I was quite happy for him to do it [*for his son to be referred*] just in case he did have some sort of, you know, congenital problem . . . well if he was being tested, fine, at least we'd get it sorted out earlier rather than later. **Ross**

The parents were also concerned about their children coming up to school age and this meant they wanted to move ahead quickly with referral:

> I sort of kept thinking like 'Oh God, school's gonna be coming up' and you know, that's what really worries me is school, I think. How he's going to cope with school. **Amy**

> We just wanted to get something done as soon as we could, I mean, certainly before he went to school 'cos I mean that would just be awful. **Gary**

'You worry, don't you?': negative feelings about referral

As well as being glad and relieved about referral, it was also possible for the parents to feel concerned and anxious about their child's referral. This was especially true where the children were experiencing other developmental difficulties and were being seen by other professionals. Fiona describes how she was waiting for an appointment to find out whether her little boy had a hearing loss due to glue ear. She wanted him referred to speech and language therapy because she was worried his problems with talking might not have been due to the hearing difficulties at all:

> Yes, he was having hearing tests . . . we didn't really know whether it was glue ear or not, and if it wasn't then I wanted to do something, you know, get moving rather than waiting all this time for appointments to come up but it might not have been that at all.

For some parents, referral meant that their worst fears about their child's diagnosis might be confirmed. At the back of their minds was the worry that the difficulties might result from a physical or general learning problem:

> That's always what worries parents. Is it something up here [*points to his head*] that isn't quite functioning right? **Ross**

Referral meant that 'something was wrong' with the child and this was very upsetting for the parents, especially where they felt the child did have a serious difficulty:

> I felt a bit worried I suppose. 'Cos if anything's wrong with your child you worry, don't you? **Amy**

> I suppose initially I was a bit shocked. I wondered whether, is there something wrong. **Emma**

Some parents also explained that having a child referred to speech and language therapy can be a stigmatizing experience. As Carol's words show, her son's referral was a traumatic event for her:

> I felt awful because, God, what will people say?

Another parent recalled how she had felt when her eldest child had been referred:

> You know, at first I thought it's like, well, a deformity, you know, I thought, 'Ooh, he's never going to be able to speak properly.' **Patricia**

When referral to speech and language therapy was necessary, a number of parents felt as if they and their children were being singled out. Their sense of loneliness and isolation was increased if they knew few other parents whose children were having similar difficulties and they felt their child was quite far behind his or her friends:

> 'Til you probably got a child with a problem you don't know anyone else who has . . . that's what makes me feel a little bit isolated and think why him . . . I know there's a lot of children who got speech problems . . . I didn't know anybody who has apart from one person. **Linda**

It was possible for the parents to experience negative feelings about referral to speech and language therapy, even when they wanted it to happen. It was also possible for them not to want their child to be referred to speech and language therapy at all. Sandra's account in Box 2.2 illustrates the fears parents might have about involving professionals and why they might be opposed to referral.

Box 2.2

Sandra had three children - a daughter aged ten, a son aged four and another son who was a toddler at the time of the interview. She recounted how her health visitor had been concerned a few years before about whether her daughter was developing a squint. The health visitor was worried that Sandra's little boy would also develop a squint. In both cases, the health visitor's concerns were investigated and proved wrong. Later on, the health visitor mentioned that Sandra's son's speech seemed to be unclear and that she was thinking of referring him to a speech and language therapist. Sandra did not feel concerned about him and felt that while he was slow in developing his speech he would eventually catch up. Having had the experience of the false alarm over her children's vision, she was reluctant for him to be referred:

> I kind of felt a bit as if, 'Oh God this again' when the speech [*when the health visitor was concerned about her son's talking*] . . . it's gonna be a yet another repetition of something that ends up to be nothing . . . I said 'No speech therapy' at first.

Eventually the referral did go ahead, at the request of the health visitor, and Sandra began to start questioning whether her child had a serious difficulty she had not been told about:

> She [*the health visitor*] sort of felt . . . that it was better to investigate it than let it be, as if there might have been a problem there.

Sandra felt that there is a tendency for professionals to become over-involved in children's early development so that no possible problems are missed. She felt that the close monitoring of her son's speech was very different from the attention he would have received in other circumstances:

> Everything gets investigated even if there wasn't, isn't a problem, doesn't it, just so that nobody's overlooked but it seems like a lot of children go through a lot just for a couple [*children who may have a real problem*] to make sure they weren't overlooked but they might get overlooked anyway. They might be in a travellers' camp or something and move on.

Sandra did not reject altogether the idea of her son being referred to speech and language therapy but she did not want it to happen so early on. Unlike the other parents, she had made the decision that she would seek help for him if the difficulties were still present when he went to school:

> He was allowed to have, be a bit slow if he wanted to be but then the independence of school I wanted it be OK by then. That was my deadline.

As these parents have shown, acknowledging that their children were having difficulties with speech and language and getting something done about the difficulties stirred up a mixture of feelings. On the one hand, the parents were pleased that professional help was available to them. On the other hand, referral to speech and language therapy was a difficult, and sometimes fearful, process for the parents to come to terms with. Certain factors seemed to make the experience more anxious for parents and increase the concern they were already feeling. These are displayed in Box 2.3.

BOX 2.3 WHAT FACTORS MADE THE PARENTS MORE ANXIOUS ABOUT REFERRAL TO SPEECH AND LANGUAGE THERAPY?

Where parents think the child has a serious difficulty.

Where the child is lagging far behind his/her friends.

Where the child has other problems with development, such as hearing loss.

Where parents feel stigmatized by the referral.

Where the child is coming up to school age.

Where parents have had no previous experience of speech and language therapy.

The parents' previous experiences

For most of the parents, this was their first experience of early speech and language difficulties and having a child referred to speech and language therapy services. Where the parents had not had any previous contact with speech and language therapy or did not know anyone else who had, being referred could be a lonely and frightening experience. Until her little boy had speech problems, no one in Carol's family had been referred to speech and language therapy. Her statement shows how difficult this process was for her:

> Well, at first I thought it was awful. At the very first . . . because . . . it's never happened to our family before, nobody else has ever been referred or anything like that and his sister was no problem at all.

Emma had had no previous experience of speech and language therapy when her daughter was referred at two-and-a-half. She explained how this affected her:

> No, I've never come across it [*speech and language therapy*] before so I suppose it was . . . quite frightening when you don't really know what's happening.

A number of parents wished that they had had the chance to meet other parents of children who had already been referred to speech and language therapy, as they felt this contact would have been helpful.

In the interviews some parents mentioned that they had already had some contact with speech and language therapy services. One mother was familiar with speech and language therapy because she worked in the field of child health and generally knew what to expect of therapy. Some parents remembered that children in their extended family had attended speech and language therapy but did not have very much knowledge about what had actually taken place. Other parents had experienced speech and language therapy in their own childhood. Selina attended speech and language therapy herself as a schoolgirl for work on the pronunciation of speech sounds. Selina's daughter's communication difficulties went hand-in-hand with a hearing loss, which meant that she was using very few words. Because of her own experience, Selina was confused about what speech and language therapy could do for her little girl:

> Well . . . I used to have speech therapy in school . . . so I was quite puzzled when they said she could have speech therapy . . . so I don't really know what it would involve 'cos in school it was like looking at the letters and trying to pronounce them.

However, the experience which appeared to have the biggest effect on the parents' feelings about their child's referral was having already gone through referral with another child. Bernadette and Ross, whose son was referred for speech difficulties when he was three-and-a-half, had visited a speech and language therapist with their daughter who had also experienced speech difficulties as a toddler. Dorothy's son was referred to speech and language therapy at three years of age. She had an older boy who had been seen by a speech and language therapist when he went to school. Where parents had already come into contact with speech and language therapy, they seemed to be less anxious about the process, as Patricia's account in Box 2.4 illustrates.

Box 2.4

Patricia had three sons who were all referred to speech and language therapy. She described how she felt when her third boy was referred:

> Well, I was quite used to it really 'cos my other two boys went.

She explained that she had found it much more difficult when her first son had been referred:

> It was more of a shock when my first one went really . . . it was all new to
> me then and like I can remember getting so upset.

Patricia also explained that she had felt stigmatized by her first
experience of referral but that this was not now a problem for her:

> From my experience with my third son I wasn't bothered at all by it, not at
> all, but I can understand it, 'cos maybe I was a little bit with my first boy,
> you know the first time, and all that, you know, not exactly going to go and
> tell everybody that he needs to see a speech therapist . . . but for how I feel
> now, quite confident about it all, so no, I wouldn't bat an eyelid really.

Because of her previous experiences, Patricia assumed that what had
been done for her two older children would be the same for the third:

> Well, I just assumed it would be the same as the other two. I did wonder a
> little bit first how he would cope with it because he always seemed,
> seemed a little bit younger in his ways than the other two.

Parents' feelings about their child's referral to speech and language therapy
were greatly influenced by their previous experience. Parents with no
previous knowledge of speech and language therapy, like Carol and Emma,
often felt concerned and alone, while parents with other children who had
attended, like Patricia, had strong ideas about what would happen. After the
referral had been made, the parents waited for their child's first appointment.
During this time there was chance for parents' expectations of speech and
language therapy to develop and take shape.

The parents' expectations of speech and language therapy

For the parents who were experiencing referral to speech and language
therapy for the first time, their main concerns were what the therapist would
be like and how formal the speech and language therapy clinic would be. A
number of parents had the idea that speech and language therapy would be
similar to other education settings. They imagined that therapy would be in
the form of school lessons and that the therapist would be a figure of
authority, like a teacher:

> I think I thought that . . . it was going to sort of be a classroom environment and it
> was going to be that she was going to sit there and be taught. **Emma**

I've never done this before and didn't know how it was going to be . . . you didn't get somebody who was sat there and was very sour . . . I thought what's this all about . . . hope that person's OK. **Carol**

I didn't know what to imagine, what would happen, how she'd be assessed, nothing at all . . . I didn't honestly know what . . . it was going to be like. Or the teacher. **Hayley**

Before attending speech and language therapy for the first time, some parents wondered what therapy activities might be like. Parents had few ideas of what would be done, although one parent who had a relative with dyslexia had imagined that speech and language therapy might follow similar lines:

My brother had dyslexia and so he had a lot of . . . exercises that he had to do with cards. **Fiona**

Some parents saw speech and language therapy as being comparable with elocution and had imagined that therapy would focus on activities to do with the pronunciation of speech sounds:

I didn't have any knowledge of what it was gonna be like so I thought obviously that they'd be concentrating on his speech . . . I wasn't very clear on how they were going to do that. **Caroline**

I thought it would be more sort of elocution-orientated . . . and I thought it would be . . . getting him used to his sounds and because . . . there was certain sounds that he totally avoided saying. **Sandra**

Well I thought they'd actually sit there . . . but like he can't say his 's's and his 'f's, sort of getting him to say 'sssock' but there wasn't none of that like. **Dorothy**

Patricia and Bernadette had both been to speech and language therapy with their older children. They imagined that therapy would be similar to what they had received previously and would take place about as often:

I could remember my other boys were going quite regularly for quite a while. **Patricia**

I mean with his sister when she had to go and it was every week she had to go. **Bernadette**

At this stage, some parents had ideas about how they, along with the therapist, would be carrying out therapy with their child:

> I knew what a speech therapist does and I know they offer the advice and . . . I'd carry it on at home as well. **Sally**

> It would be something maybe I'd carry on at home but that I'd be given ideas or tasks or, you know, little project things to do with him in the time that we worked on and then we'd look at how he'd done then when we went back. **Caroline**

Waiting for the first appointment

The children of the parents who took part in the interviews were referred to one of two speech and language therapy services. Very often, the parents mentioned that their health visitors had warned them in advance that they might face a long wait for their first appointment. However, these parents reported that their waiting times were between one and four months, which was acceptable to them. The parents felt that the wait for an appointment at speech and language therapy was much shorter than that for other hospital departments. Fiona waited for an appointment for her son to see the ear, nose and throat consultant at the hospital and this made the speech and language therapy waiting time seem very short in comparison:

> It wasn't very long at all . . . maybe a couple of months I guess, but having waited for a year for his appointment with the hospital, that was marvellous.

During the waiting period, unless the parents had had some previous contact with speech and language therapy, they could only imagine what might happen when they attended for the first time. The next chapter explores what happened when the parents first attended speech and language therapy for their child and their reactions to it.

Summary of the chapter

- For their child to be referred to speech and language therapy, the parents approached their health visitor or GP or made the referral themselves.
- Generally the parents felt uncertain about whether their child was experiencing real difficulties. However, there is research which suggests that parents can be good judges of whether there is a problem with their children's speech and language development.
- On the whole the parents were positive about referral but also experienced feelings of concern and anxiety. One parent was very unhappy about her son being referred.

- The parents felt less anxious about attending speech and language therapy if they had had other recent experiences of it.
- While they were waiting for their first appointment, the parents were anxious about what speech and language therapy would be like.
- The parents recalled that the waiting time between the referral being made and their first appointment was between one and four months.

CHAPTER 3

The first visit to speech and language therapy

When the parents were sure that their children's difficulties with talking were not improving, many were very eager for their child to be seen by a speech and language therapist. All of the parents who took part in the interviews had first visited speech and language therapy more than 12 months before. In spite of the length of time in between, many of the parents were able to recall what had happened and what they had been told when they had their first appointment. Even clearer were their memories of how they felt at that time. In this chapter, the parents' accounts of their first visit to speech and language therapy will be considered in detail. The features of the first appointment recalled by the parents are listed in Box 3.1.

BOX 3.1 FEATURES OF THEIR FIRST APPOINTMENT RECALLED BY THE PARENTS

The length of the appointment.

What the child, parents and therapist did in the appointment.

The explanations given about the child's difficulties during the appointment.

The advice given to parents about helping their child's talking in the appointment.

How parents felt about the first appointment.

The length of the first appointment

When parents bring their children to speech and language therapy initially, the speech and language therapist will carry out a detailed assessment of the child's speech and language skills. This may involve the therapist looking at pictures with the child, asking the child questions and observing the child at

28

play. The therapist may also ask parents questions about other aspects of the child's development and behaviour, hearing, medical history and whether there have been similar problems in the family before. This process takes time as the therapist will be trying to find out more about the child's difficulties and to decide what should be done about them. The parents who were interviewed felt that this assessment process was quite long, usually about one to one-and-a-half hours. For some parents, the appointments had been broken down into shorter, and more manageable, chunks of time, such as 30 to 35 minutes. The parents recognized that the therapist needed time to be able to do the assessment. However, they felt that long appointments were a problem if their child became bored or upset and if a brother or sister was present who needed their attention:

> It felt a long time in the actual assessment but probably it was only about an hour, an hour-and-a-half . . . I remember her younger brother and he was getting very fractious and I remember thinking but you know I think it was the right amount of time. **Emma**

> So it was OK. I suppose I would have thought it was too long if he was like wanting to go or not listening. **Caroline**

On the whole, the parents did not feel that the time taken to assess their child caused too many problems. One mother was surprised that so much time was spent assessing her little boy and was pleased to think that the therapist was doing a thorough assessment:

> It was very good . . . we were in there for an hour at least, a good hour and that was brilliant because . . . a lot of time is spent with him. **Carol**

Other parents thought that the assessment time needed to be long so that their child could get used to being in the clinic and cooperate better with what the therapist was trying to do:

> It seemed to need that long . . . to get him into the idea of what she [*the therapist*] needed him to do anyway. **Patricia**

The parents, also, felt that they needed time, particularly where the time leading up to the first appointment had been anxious:

> I think that's what's needed to give yourself time to get in there to unwind and to let the child relax enough to assess her. **Emma**

What the child, parents and therapist did

When they thought back over their first appointment at speech and language therapy, the parents explained that the therapist needed to build up a picture of their child's skills during this session. They recalled activities like playing with their child, the therapist asking the child questions and looking at pictures in a book with the child and being asked questions themselves by the therapist:

> She [*the therapist*] listened to him and . . . just asked me questions . . . I know he had a game . . . he had a car and to see his imagination, imaginary play, what he would say. **Linda**

> She [*the therapist*] went through the book and spoke to him about various different pictures, played puzzle games with him . . . and then we sat down and had a play afterwards. **Fiona**

> She [*the therapist*] sat and asked me what I thought his problems were and I told her and then she spent some time trying to get him to say pictures and things like that. **Dorothy**

One mother who had training in child care and development reported which areas of the child's development the therapist had tested out – his understanding of language, his imaginary play and his speech sounds:

> He done quite well at that 'cos he's got very good understanding . . . and then he spent about . . . ten minutes or so actually playing with me on the floor, sort of imaginary play . . . the sounds of the words I think was what they were trying to pick up on initially. **Sally**

Some parents were given an explanation by the therapist they saw about what activities were being carried out and the reasons for them. Where parents had received an explanation they found it easier to recall those activities. For some parents, however, there was some confusion and misunderstanding about what the therapist was trying to find out, especially if the purpose of certain activities had not been explained to them. In a number of cases, this led to the parents questioning some assessment activities. Caroline's account in Box 3.2 shows how parents may come to doubt whether some activities are helpful.

On the whole the parents were happy with the activities that took place as part of the assessment. While some parents showed uncertainty about particular activities, such as the testing of speech sounds in Caroline's case, for many of the parents the activities appeared to make sense:

They seemed like normal assessments, seemed quite logical to me, going through and checking out how he was responding to different questions. **Fiona**

Box 3.2

Caroline's small son first attended speech and language therapy when he was about two years old. At the time he was saying only a few words. A particular aspect of children's communication skills which may be targeted in the assessment process is their speech sound system. To test this area in Caroline's child, a number of objects were presented to him for him to name, so that the therapist could gather information about the sounds and groups of sounds he was using. As Caroline explains:

> She [*the therapist*] just asked him what she had there and they weren't . . .
> I didn't feel they tested his abilities very well.

Because his vocabulary was very limited, Caroline felt he should have been learning simpler words:

> Because it was sort of words that he wouldn't have come across . . . whereas he was more at the stage where he could say 'no', 'yes' and 'Mummy', 'Daddy' . . . and real basic things like that whereas I think she just concentrated mainly on objects that she had, that she wanted him to say.

The reason behind the activity was not explained to Caroline and she did not feel that the therapist could gain any useful information from asking her son to name objects and that he would not benefit from it.

The parents also described a number of other positive aspects of the assessment activities. Where the atmosphere of the appointment had been relaxed, the parents felt that this had put the children at ease and helped them to cooperate with the activities. The parents were pleased when they found that the materials used by the therapist in the assessment process included toys the children had already come across and enjoyed playing with. For parents whose children are experiencing difficulties with early language learning, there is a tendency, perhaps, to focus on the areas of development where the problems are and to see the child in terms of the things he or she is not able to do. For this reason, the parents felt very positively about the situations and activities in their first appointment where the children did well and were able to show their strengths. Also, in a number of cases the parents found it helpful to watch how the therapist interacted with their child. From this they felt that they gained ideas which they could try out away from the speech and language therapy clinic.

There were, however, some aspects of the assessment which parents were less happy about. As Caroline's explanation showed, she felt that the therapist her son saw used a test which did not take his small vocabulary into account. To her, this part of the assessment had seemed pointless. Another mother was concerned about the way in which tests have to be carried out with children. Sandra's little boy failed some questions which she thought he should have passed. This happened because the therapist had to ask the question in a standard way and this meant using vocabulary her son did not know. The positive and negative aspects of the assessment activities are summarized in Box 3.3.

Box 3.3

Positive aspects of assessment activities recalled by the parents

The relaxed nature of the assessment time helped the child to join in:

> I felt that it was nice and relaxed because she definitely felt quite comfortable and she was actually able to be observed. **Emma**

Many of the toys used in the assessment were familiar to the child:

> I mean the cards what they used and the toys what they had on the table were all sort of toys like what was around the house so it wasn't going to be difficult for him to say. **Bernadette**

The activities showed what the child *could* do:

> He is good at sitting down and doing that sort of thing so . . . yeah, it was fine. **Andrea**

The activities could be picked up on and tried out at home:

> I think that's what helped me when I got home to think . . . this is what she needs . . . it's nice to actually see how somebody else sort of has a go at something. **Emma**

Negative aspects of assessment activities recalled by parents

The use of tests which parents felt did not take the child's stage of development into account:

> I just felt it didn't really look at him as what he could do and so progress
> with him. **Caroline**

The use of tests which have to be carried out in a particular way:

> I mean she [*the therapist*] knew that she had to say it in a certain way . . .
> some mothers use different terminology for different things so it might not
> be something your child relates to but it was the standard . . . test. **Sandra**

The explanations given about the child's difficulties

For the parents the most important part of their first visit to speech and
language therapy was the chance to find out if there was a problem with their
child's speech and language and to see what could be done about it. Linked
very closely with this idea was the parents' hope that they would receive an
explanation of the problem. As Chapter 1 showed, very often the parents had
their own ideas about what the problem was and possible causes. By
attending speech and language therapy, they hoped to find out more about
the difficulties. In the interviews, the parents recalled varying types of explanation of the difficulties given them by the speech and language therapist
they saw, listed in Box 3.4.

Box 3.4 EXPLANATIONS OF THE CHILD'S DIFFICULTIES RECALLED BY THE
PARENTS

Descriptive explanations.

Explanations about cause.

Explanations involving advice.

General explanations.

Firstly, some parents remembered that the speech and language therapist had
explained the difficulties to them by describing what was happening in their
child's speech. Sometimes the therapist would pinpoint the sounds the child
was not using or was not able to pronounce correctly and explain why
certain sounds caused problems for young children:

> But obviously he wasn't just pronouncing some of the words, which letters, it was
> particular letters that it had been tied to. **Ross**

I mean his first problem at the time was . . . she [*the therapist*] thought he never had no endings on any of his words. **Amy**

Secondly, other parents felt that they had been given an explanation about why the difficulties had arisen and what factors were interfering with their child developing language normally:

Because of her hearing loss she was not catching on as quick as other children. That was the only thing they could explain why she was like she was. **Selina**

I think they would have mentioned that it does sort of tend to happen quite a lot where the older one will do the work for the younger one and the younger one seems quite happy to sort of sit back and let him. Yeah, that's the only explanation I think. **Wendy**

I mean there was, you know, a little bit of doubt as to whether it could still be something physical because she hadn't long had her adenoids removed at that point. **Isabel**

Thirdly, a few parents reported that the explanations given to them by the speech and language therapist involved advice and overlapped with ideas about what would help particular difficulties:

I mean I was given a list of suggestions of areas I could work on . . . certain sounds he had trouble with and making a scrapbook up of the sounds he was having. **Sally**

Fourthly, some parents pointed out that the speech and language therapist had given more general explanations of the difficulties by linking them with other developmental skills:

She [*the therapist*] was saying 'cos he was quite slow with his eating of solid foods and she was explaining that sometimes means that they're going to be slower with their speech 'cos they haven't formed all their muscles properly or something and aren't used to using them in that way. **Caroline**

I think they just said it's mostly to do with like her concentration . . . just trying to get her to listen really. **Monica**

Several parents felt that they had never been given explanations for the difficulties at all, even though their child's areas of weakness had been identified:

No one knew, told me why. I mean we all knew he couldn't talk but why can't he talk? This is what I didn't get an answer for and even today I haven't really got an answer for why he can't do it. **Linda**

I can't remember the reasons as to why there was perhaps a delay. I don't think that somebody mentioned that. **Emma**

Not actually explanations . . . I think, I don't know we know really at the moment why . . . he has had a difficulty. **Carol**

One mother had been told that there were no known reasons for early difficulties:

She [*the therapist*] did say . . . that there is no particular reason or they don't know of any particular reason. **Kate**

For other parents, the need to get an explanation for their child's difficulties was not a pressing one. Patricia had three sons all of whom were referred to speech and language therapy. She recalled having been told by the therapist who saw her second child that although her two elder children had experienced difficulties, this did not mean that any other child she had would also have difficulties. The therapist informed her that problems existed in children on an individual basis and a history of difficulties in the family would not make a difference to her third son. Perhaps for that reason Patricia was not as concerned as other parents to find an answer:

I didn't really realize, know why there is a reason. I thought it was just an individual thing . . . just because one child has it doesn't mean your next child's gonna get it.

Fiona had been anxious for her son to be referred to speech and language therapy. His hearing was being checked at that time and she wanted to make sure that his language difficulties were not being caused by something else. She was convinced, however, that the hearing difficulties had been at the root of the problem with talking and, like Patricia, was not anxious to get an explanation. When she was asked if she had received an explanation about the difficulties she responded that she had told the speech and language therapist her own views:

I think I gave why I thought he had difficulties, from the other way round.

The advice given to parents

All the parents interviewed talked about the advice they had received from the speech and language therapist they had seen. Parents could remember two main types of advice given by the therapist during the initial visit, as shown in Box 3.5.

Box 3.5 Types of advice recalled by the parents

Advice tied to particular problems, especially difficulties with speech sounds.

General advice to encourage language development.

A number of parents were given specific information about dealing with specific difficulties. When their children were experiencing difficulties with speech sounds, a few parents mentioned being advised by the therapist to repeat a word back to their child after he or she had said it incorrectly:

And always correct him the once and then leave it. **Bernadette**

He says something to me, I repeat it back to him the proper way. **Carol**

Just to sort of repeat . . . it so if he said it and it wasn't correct that I would just sort of say, 'Oh you want a drink, do you?' **Caroline**

Other parents remembered the therapist advising them not to ask their child questions so much. Where they did need to question the child, they were shown how to make it easier for the child to respond by using closed questions such as, 'Do you want milk or water?' rather than open questions such as, 'What do you want to drink?':

I know that I was told perhaps not to question so much . . . perhaps to just sit there and I know that I was asking open questions to her and she just wasn't capable of doing it. **Emma**

Several parents of children who had speech sound problems recalled being told by the therapist to discourage their child's use of a dummy or bottle or to cut out their use altogether:

She [*the therapist*] just suggested that perhaps if we could cut him down using it, it would help. **Ross**

It's what I was told was causing his problem with his 's's and that lot because sucking on the bottle. **Dorothy**

A number of other parents were given more general advice about helping their children to develop their language skills. This often took the form of practical ideas to try out with the child during the time they spent at home together. This advice included encouraging the child to make eye contact when talking:

> She [*the therapist*] wanted me to direct it at him more but then I think you naturally do that anyway, if a child's not concentrating on you, you do tend to grab him gently by the shoulders . . . and direct him in your face. **Sandra**

A few parents remembered the therapist explaining how to help their child to focus on one activity at a time by telling them to take away things that distracted the child, particularly while he or she was playing:

> We bought a lot of toys for her . . . so we was told to pack them up and put them away . . . because too much of the same thing they just lose interest quickly. **Selina**

Some other parents recalled being encouraged by the therapist to look at books with their child more and to play games where the child needed to use language:

> It was just like try the games . . . and sit and read to her. **Hayley**

> It's like playing games with him and getting him to say like the things you were playing with. **Dorothy**

While parents felt that some of the advice they were given was common sense they also felt that some of the advice had contained ideas they would not have thought of for themselves:

> It [*the advice from the therapist*] steered me into the path that I obviously should be taking which I wouldn't have had. **Emma**

> Some ideas that she was giving me I don't think I would ever have thought of really, you know, even though they were common sense things. **Patricia**

More than a year on from their first visit to speech and language therapy, some parents commented how the ideas they were given have become a part of the routine and now take place as an accepted part of everyday life:

> I mean it's become a habit, the natural thing to do with him. He says something to me, I repeat it back to him the proper way . . . it's second nature . . . it's not a problem it's . . . a way of life really. **Carol**

In general, the parent felt that the advice they had been given by the speech and language therapist at the first visit was helpful. As this mother explained, the ideas she received early on were to be the most positive aspect of her whole experience of speech and language therapy for her little boy:

> She [*the therapist*] just really . . . emphasized some things that I could do myself with him just to help him along a bit and that was the only thing I really got out of it, the whole thing, and I'm sure he really didn't get anything out of it, as such, except for I could perhaps put in practice what she had said to me. **Sandra**

However, other parents were not so positive about the advice they had been given. In particular, the parents did not feel reassured about carrying out advice if it was something they felt they were doing automatically or already doing without any effects being felt. One mother expressed her unhappiness about the lack of fresh ideas to try out with her son:

> It's what you do with your kids anyway, it's like when you read books to them, you get them to try and copy the words like. **Dorothy**

She did not feel that what she was already doing was enough as her little boy was still making little progress and she had expected to receive more information from the therapist. There were also instances where the parents felt awkward and inadequate about advice given by the therapist. One parent remembered that she had been advised to buy certain games for her child, which, as a single parent, she knew she was unable to afford:

> She [*the therapist*] told me to get some games . . . but the thing is when you're on your own bringing them up, you haven't got that money to go and get every game that they want you to get. **Hayley**

Another mother felt that the advice given her by the therapist was not information she could benefit from but more of a personal criticism of the way she was coping with her son's talking difficulties:

> I suppose she [*the therapist*] did have some points but I just thought . . . I think I felt like I was being told off rather than educated . . . rather than her saying it was her opinion, that was what she thought, it was like, no . . . this is it . . . I did sort of feel that she just wasn't giving me an idea or an area to work towards, it was a bit sort of, a telling off. **Caroline**

How the parents felt about the first appointment

After the early concerns they had about their children's talking, their contact with the health visitor and the wait for referral to speech and language therapy, the first visit to speech and language therapy often came as something of a relief to the parents. At this point, they were able to find out more about their child's difficulties, observe how their child got on within the assessment situation and receive explanations and advice. For many of the parents the first appointment at speech and language therapy turned out to be quite different from what they had expected. In some cases, they were pleasantly surprised that visiting speech and language therapy had been a fairly relaxed experience and that their appointment had gone well. Other parents were less satisfied with the activities and advice which had been part of this first visit. When the parents were interviewed over a year on, memories of their initial appointment had receded and some aspects of it were only partly recalled. Very often, however, the parents were able to discuss the visit in terms of their feelings about it and highlighted both positive and negative aspects of their attendance at speech and language therapy. Both aspects are summarized in Box 3.6.

Box 3.6

Positive aspects of the first attendance at speech and language therapy

Where they already had experienced speech and language therapy, the parents tended to feel confident about attending.

The parents felt pleased if their child coped well with the assessment process.

The parents found it comforting if the therapist could not discover any specific physical or mental basis for their child's difficulties.

When the therapist's description of the child's difficulties agreed with their own, the parents were reassured.

The parents were happy when they were able to get ideas from watching the therapist working with the child.

The parents were glad that the assessment process showed up other areas where the child was having difficulties such as problems with understanding.

The parents' initial feelings of shock and fear of the unknown were replaced by feelings of reassurance and confidence.

The parents felt that their decision to seek referral was justified when the difficulties were confirmed by the therapist and that others could no longer dismiss the child's problems.

The parents felt that others involved with their child would try to be more understanding because the difficulties were confirmed.

The parents enjoyed the positive interaction between them, their child and the therapist.

The parents were pleased to receive feedback from the assessment and to know how their children were getting on.

Negative aspects of the first attendance at speech and language therapy

The parents could often be very nervous about attending speech and language therapy and what the diagnosis might be.

The parents sometimes felt that the therapist viewed their child negatively.

The parents were unhappy when they did not receive an explanation of the problem or where they were not completely sure whether there was a problem or not.

The parents often worried about how they and their child would get on with the therapist.

The parents were concerned that speech and language therapy might be too strict for their children.

Sometimes the parents felt that the assessment process was not tailored to suit the individual child.

The parents were doubtful about how useful some of the assessment tasks were.

At the first visit the therapist used the time to assess the child and talk to the parents. When this process was completed, the parents were keen to learn from the therapist what the problem with their child's talking was. At assessment, the children of all the parents who were interviewed as part of this project were experiencing notable difficulties with speech and language. Their parents were eager to find out what would then happen and it is this aspect which will be explored in the next chapter.

Summary of the chapter

- Parents recalled a number of aspects of their first visit to speech and language therapy, including the length of the appointment, what happened in the session, the explanations given about their child's difficulties and advice about helping their child.
- Generally the parents were satisfied with the way in which their child had been assessed by the speech and language therapist but were concerned that some of the tasks used might be unfair to the child.
- Some of the parents remembered being given some explanation of their child's difficulties by the therapist.
- The parents were also given advice about dealing with the child's specific difficulties and generally promoting their child's language development.
- The parents expressed a mixture of positive and negative views of their first attendance at speech and language therapy but on the whole were eager to move forward following the assessment.

Chapter 4

Considering the options in speech and language therapy

At the end of their child's first visit to speech and language therapy, the parents were concerned to do something to address the difficulties the therapist had identified. In many speech and language therapy departments at this point, the speech and language therapist would discuss with parents what options existed for therapy and a way forward would be decided upon. Dependent upon the speech and language therapy department visited and the nature of the child's difficulties, several different courses of action might be possible. These are illustrated in Box 4.1.

Box 4.1 Possibilities for the form of speech and language therapy for pre-school children

Review

If the therapist identifies that the child has difficulties but judges that they are either likely to start improving by themselves or that therapy would not be appropriate at that time, the child might be put on review. This means that the child will not start receiving therapy straightaway but will be invited back after a period of time (usually three to six months) for the therapist to re-assess and check on the progress made. Therapy may or may not be viewed as necessary at the end of the review period.

Therapy

The therapist judges that the child's difficulties are unlikely to start improving without help and that it is appropriate for treatment to begin. Speech and language therapy might then be offered in the form of:

- Individual therapy for the child's difficulties, where the child is seen by the therapist, usually with the parent(s) present

---

- Group therapy for the child's difficulties, where the child receives treatment in a group with children who have similar problems
- Therapy in the form of a programme drawn up by the therapist to be carried out by others involved with the children, for example, nursery staff
- Therapy in the form of a group offered to the parents to give them ways to help their child's speech and language development
- A combination of any of the above approaches.

However, the experience of the parents whose stories are told in this book was slightly different from this. This was because they had given consent for their children to take part in a research project, which decided for them which treatment option their child would receive. In this chapter, the parents talk about their experiences of the treatment options in the project and discuss the advantages and disadvantages of the options.

About the research project

This project was designed to compare the progress of children who received speech and language therapy at the local community clinic immediately following assessment with that of children whose therapy was delayed for 12 months. The project aimed to answer two main questions, shown in Box 4.2.

BOX 4.2 WHAT THE PROJECT WAS AIMING TO FIND OUT

Did children who received therapy immediately improve more than children who didn't?

Did the children whose therapy was delayed get better on their own?

Instead of the therapist and the parents discussing and deciding how therapy would take place, the parents allowed their children to be allocated to immediate or delayed therapy on the basis of chance. This was done by the parents opening an envelope containing the allocation. Neither the parents nor the therapist knew in advance what the allocation would be. Altogether, 159 children took part in the research. Thus, within the context of the project, after they had been assessed, there were two possibilities regarding what would happen next to the children, as Box 4.3 shows.

Box 4.3 WHAT HAPPENED TO THE CHILDREN IN THE PROJECT?

Immediate therapy

They started receiving therapy straight away and were then re-assessed after six and then 12 months. Altogether, 71 of the 159 children were allocated to this group. The children were seen individually by the speech and language therapist usually with their parent(s) present. The actual treatment they received was exactly the same as what would have been offered to any other children coming for individual therapy for the same difficulties.

Therapy later

Their difficulties were monitored and their parents received advice to help them facilitate their child's speech and language development. This group of children were also re-assessed after six (at which point parents might opt to join the immediate therapy group) and then 12 months. A total of 88 children were allocated to this group. This approach is similar to the child being put on review. If the children were still experiencing difficulties at the end of their time in the project, they received an intensive course of therapy from speech and language therapists involved in the research.

Following their allocation, both groups of children were seen for re-assessment six months after their first assessment and another six months after that. The parents were free to withdraw their child from the project at any point. Also, if the parents of children who came into the delayed therapy group decided at any time during the 12 months that they wanted to start receiving treatment for their child they could do so. Even though the children were participating in a research project, the options within the project – having immediate access to therapy or delaying therapy – are not too different from what might be offered in everyday service settings where research is not taking place. Therefore, it is relevant to examine how the parents felt about the option they were offered – immediate or delayed treatment.

Exploring the parents' views of immediate treatment *versus* waiting

To find out how the parents felt about receiving treatment straightaway or delaying therapy and how the children progressed in these two groups, the interviews were designed to include parents whose children had received immediate therapy and also parents whose children had waited. Of the 20 interviews which are reported on in this book, six of them were with parents of children who received therapy immediately, another six were with parents of children whose therapy was delayed and a further eight were with parents of children originally allocated to delayed therapy but who opted for them to start receiving treatment.

All of the parents interviewed spoke at length of their views about the therapy option they were offered. They were often able to recall how they had felt about their child being allocated to immediate or delayed therapy at the beginning of their involvement in the project. They also expressed their views about the effects the therapy option had had on them, their child and their family during their participation in the research. Over the whole course of their involvement in the project, some of the parents preferred to receive intervention immediately, while other parents were happier to delay it. Both options were acceptable to differing sets of parents, depending upon a number of factors. In terms of their satisfaction with the therapy option they received, it was possible to divide the parents into a number of groups, as Box 4.4 shows.

BOX 4.4 SATISFACTION OF THE PARENTS WITH THE THERAPY OPTION RECEIVED

Satisfied with receiving therapy immediately.

Dissatisfied with receiving therapy immediately.

Satisfied with delaying therapy.

Dissatisfied with delaying therapy.

Satisfaction with receiving therapy immediately

Amy, Selina and Patricia all felt that receiving treatment immediately would be beneficial to their children. In the interviews, they expressed the sense of relief they felt at getting the 'right envelope' – being allocated to the option they wanted, as their statements show:

> I was a bit worried, I must admit if he hadn't got on the project [*been allocated to immediate treatment*] I'd have been really worried. **Amy**

> I was pleased that she got the . . . option where she had it [*therapy*] intensely. I was very concerned if we pulled the other envelope. **Selina**

I thought it was good really. I thought that was the lucky envelope in a way.
Patricia

All three mothers also described how they felt their child needed help at that
point. They felt that their progress might have been put at risk if they had had
to wait for treatment and so were keen for therapy to begin:

So I think if he'd have been left it would have been another year . . . but he
wouldn't get there on his own, he definitely wouldn't. **Amy**

I was relieved that she was going to get the attention that I thought she needed.
Selina

So I thought if I don't get therapy now . . . he's just left, he's left to me . . . so yeah I
was pleased really that . . . he was getting help. **Patricia**

Amy felt that the therapy her son had received for his speech sound difficulties had worked for him and helped him to move on. She also believed
that the more therapy he received, the better the progress he was able to
make:

Everything seemed to work well enough . . . every area we dealt with with him he
sort of grasped, you know . . . I just feel the more speech therapy he has, the better
he's getting.

Selina explained that therapy was available for her daughter when it was
needed and without it, she would still be struggling with her speech and
language development:

It was a great help when we needed it, I think, because if she'd been left I don't
think she would be as forward as she is.

Patricia felt that her little boy had gained from receiving therapy but also
highlighted how the therapy had helped her to have a positive effect on his
speech and language difficulties:

I was pleased, it's been good . . . I know I benefited from it, definitely, because,
you know, it helped me to help him really.

Essentially, these three mothers were happy with the help they had
been given and put their children's improvement down to the treatment they
had received.

Dissatisfaction with receiving therapy immediately

For another mother, whose child had been allocated to immediate therapy, however, having immediate access to therapy was not acceptable. Sandra, the mother who had strongly resisted referral to speech and language therapy was disappointed when her son was allocated to immediate therapy:

> I was hoping I was going to be one of the ones that could've waited . . . I was hoping I would be put on the waiting list.

Sandra's unhappiness about receiving therapy straightaway sprang from her belief that her child, given time, would get better on his own and for that reason delaying therapy was the course of action she preferred. Unlike Amy, Selina and Patricia, Sandra felt that for her son to make progress, he would be better off if given the chance to make improvement on his own:

> I was a bit gutted that it was all going ahead so soon 'cos I wanted to give him longer 'cos I thought that there might not be a problem in another six months' time . . . because six months is a long time when you're three or something isn't it?

Sandra felt that receiving therapy straight away raised real doubts for her about the progress her son was likely to make and how serious his problems were. She expressed her view that immediate therapy was harmful, because it made her begin to feel negative in her outlook on her child and his future:

> That's the damage it did, just by my attitude, thinking you know that maybe things weren't going to be alright . . . it made me feel as if there was something wrong with him, you know, gave me different insight to him which I didn't want to see.

Eventually Sandra decided to stop attending therapy altogether. Given the choice, it is clear that Sandra would have preferred to delay therapy. As well as having doubts about whether immediate therapy was the right approach for her little boy, Sandra's family circumstances became very difficult during this time:

> It was bad timing, it was a very bad time in my life and I suppose I didn't really want to put any energy into thinking that there was anything wrong with him.

She was helping to care for a member of her family who was terminally ill and this increased responsibility made attending speech and language therapy sessions very inconvenient:

I was finding it too much [*attending speech and language therapy*] . . . partly because of what else was going on . . . but it was making me feel lower as well.

While they may not have been experiencing such difficult circumstances as Sandra, delaying therapy was a popular option among some of the parents who actually did experience it.

Satisfaction with delaying therapy

A number of parents whose children's therapy was delayed, were content with this option and explained why it was not difficult for them to wait for therapy, as Bernadette and Ross's account in Box 4.5 illustrates.

Box 4.5

Bernadette and Ross's son was first assessed by a speech and language therapist when he was three-and-a-half years old. Bernadette reported that he was making noticeable progress at this time. For that reason, they felt he would be best served by a further wait to see if the difficulties were going to get better without treatment:

> They asked if we would mind sort of like doing the programme [*taking part in the research project*] . . . what would we feel about waiting and leaving it and we [*she and the child's father, Ross*] both agreed it was alright . . . 'cos he was beginning to come on then . . . he was beginning to sort of catch up a bit.

Bernadette contrasted the experience of their son with what had happened to his elder sister. She had been referred to speech and language therapy at a similar age because her speech was unclear. She had received therapy at the local community clinic. Both Bernadette and her husband had been under the impression that their son would be offered similar care. However, when he was allocated to delayed therapy they were delighted by the difference in the way their son's difficulties were dealt with:

> It was different but I mean we were certainly happy with the difference . . . I was more than happy with it . . . the whole approach this time was completely different. It wasn't so regimented. I never felt comfortable when I used to go for the speech therapy sessions with her.

Giving their son the opportunity to develop on his own was important to them. However, they were both reassured by the fact that his

---

difficulties would be monitored on the project and that help would be available if the improvements did not continue:

> There was always . . . that safety net there knowing that if it wasn't going right or if he deteriorated along the way you knew that there was something that could be offered later.

A number of other parents were glad that they had the chance to see how their children would develop, when left to do it at their own pace. At the same time they were relieved that somebody was still keeping track of their children's difficulties:

> He's been allowed to develop as he wants but I've known that we're not out of the scheme . . . so that if I do feel there's a problem, I can do something about it . . . I knew that I was still involved, it was just we were allowing it to see what happened so I didn't feel like I'd been sort of forgotten. **Andrea**

> It was nice to let her develop . . . but to be monitored at the same time was nice. **Emma**

It became clear that, for these parents, an important part of the delayed therapy option was the regular re-assessment which took place as part of it. The first re-assessment took place after six months and the second another six months after that. All the parents felt that this was essential for reassuring them and helping them to see whether their child had made progress. They appreciated that a certain time had to elapse to make re-assessment worthwhile, as these statements reveal:

> I think if we'd had them sooner there wouldn't have been that much development with her . . . I think that the six months is the right amount of time. **Emma**

> It seemed to come round quite quickly the six months so that wasn't too long a break in between and he had plenty of time . . . to progress so there was at least a change when we went. **Andrea**

It seemed unlikely, therefore, that any of the parents would have consented to a year's wait without the knowledge that they would be seen in between:

> I don't think I would have been very happy with that [*waiting the full year without the six month re-assessment*]. **Bernadette**

While these parents were anticipating that their child's problems could get better in the course of the year, they were also reassured that help would be available if they did not. This was an important consideration for some of the parents particularly if their children might be coming up to the start of school:

Provided it progressed itself before he went to school which it has virtually, it's fine. **Bernadette**

We didn't think there was a major, major, major problem there so we didn't think things should be getting done straightaway. It was just, we wanted it watched just made sure 'cos we had the time 'til he went to school. **Ross**

It wasn't that much of a blow really because still we had that extra time because he wasn't going to school, you know, if he was going to school then I would be a bit, you know, a bit worried, more worried. **Carol**

I thought the timing was fine and I mean I was lucky in that I was sort of due to see a therapist and the timings would have been quite good because if he did need intense therapy, it would have still been, he would still have got it before he actually started school. **Wendy**

So while some of the parents agreed to a delay in therapy for their children, they were balancing this with the need for their children to be ready for entry into school, a significant event in the life of any child.

By the end of their time in the project, several of the parents were convinced that the waiting period had had positive effects. They explained that because therapy had been put on hold, when it did start, their child was able to take part in and cooperate with it better. This might not have been the case if they had started receiving it earlier:

So looking back now I was pleased those six months we did wait 'cos time he had the therapy then I think he was ready for it so yes, looking back now but at the time no, I was disappointed. **Linda**

I think if you'd put her on speech therapy earlier she may not have benefited because she wasn't ready for it whereas I think now . . . she's at the point where she's like a sponge she absorbs everything she's got patience where she would have been quite young six months ago or a year ago. **Emma**

Although this option was popular with some of the parents who experienced it, other parents were very dissatisfied.

Dissatisfaction with delaying therapy

It became evident in the course of the interviews that the two options to which the children could be allocated in the project became closely linked in the parents' minds with how likely their children were to make progress. While all parents had given their consent to participate in the project, a number of the parents described how disappointed they were in agreeing to delay therapy. They talked about how their child had been 'left' to them. At the time they believed that improvement would only come about in their children if they were to receive therapy immediately, as these parents' accounts reveal:

> Gutted . . . I mean, yeah, we were very disappointed . . . it would have been a great relief to have sat there and it was therapy now . . . it would have been much better, you knew that, you knew you were going to get advice and support right from the word go as opposed to waiting. **Gary**

> I was a bit disappointed . . . he had a problem with his speech and I was a bit disappointed with that I must admit. I thought well, if he needs help I've got to wait six months now [*until the six month re-assessment*] 'til he gets it. **Linda**

Sometimes, the parents became disappointed at delaying therapy because they were struggling to cope with the difficulties that arose from the child's communication difficulties. One mother, herself a child health professional, felt inadequate to deal with the difficulties on her own without a speech and language therapist to help:

> Well, I felt that he needed help because he was just getting crosser and crosser and I mean . . . what I was doing wasn't enough and it wasn't improving and he was suffering from it. **Sally**

These parents described how they had needed to think very carefully about becoming involved in the project. It had been necessary for them to weigh up the pros and cons of taking part in the research when their consent was originally sought by the speech and language therapist. If they had particular reasons for wanting their children to make progress quickly, they found it more difficult to balance their own ideas of what their child needed with involvement in the project which might delay the help they wanted to receive.

For some parents, the option of delaying therapy interfered so much with their children's progress that they opted for their child to abandon the waiting option and start receiving treatment straightaway (Box 4.6).

Box 4.6

Linda, Hayley, Jacky and Gary, Kate, Monica and Isabel all changed option at about the six month point when their children were re-assessed, while Fiona made her decision to change about three weeks after allocation. These statements illustrate their common fear that their children were not getting better and therefore needed to start therapy:

> He was three and I think then, I mean the gap was getting wider. His speech was falling behind and I wasn't happy with that and I think he needed help so that was why I wanted to change. **Linda**

> Sort of all that we knew was that we wanted him to be better than what he was and be able to communicate and mix more confidently than what he was doing . . . so we just wanted to get something done as soon as we possibly could. **Gary**

> At that time he didn't appear to have improved. **Kate**

> I thought well really yeah, she does need help then so that's why I decided, well I can at least try and ring and say no, I'm not happy, you know, she's still doing this mumbling. **Monica**

> 'Cos there had been so little progress with the speech . . . there had been in a period of six months very little change in her speech . . . so my anxieties were raised. **Isabel**

The approach of entry into school strongly encouraged the parents to begin their children's therapy:

> It was just because there was nothing else coming, no speech coming from her . . . 'cos I thought time is going on . . . she will be going to school and I don't want her to be that far behind, behind everybody else. **Hayley**

> He needed to be on a par with his, you know, his peers . . . and there's an awful lot of things that he's got to take on board for starting school, even if he was, you know, in line with his peers let alone a year behind . . . that's a major thing that I felt we can't wait for the year. **Fiona**

In the interviews, the parents talked about their decision to start receiving speech and language therapy and why waiting was no longer acceptable. Their explanations demonstrate the sense of urgency they felt:

I thought well, he needs, he's still not talking now, he needs help. If he's going I didn't want him to feel awkward when he went to nursery so I wanted him to have some help really by then. **Linda**

I thought, 'Well, I've got to think about what's best for him' and at that time he needed help then . . . he wasn't getting involved with his peers . . . he was finding that upsetting so I couldn't justify saying OK, we'll go along with this research group and wait for a year because he needed help then. **Fiona**

'Cos I was so frantic I was determined that she was going to go back to speech therapy and have it. **Hayley**

Another factor which seemed to increase parents' anxieties about delaying therapy was a history of hearing loss or the possibility that their child was continuing to experience hearing loss. Linda's son's hearing fluctuated during the time of his involvement in the project and he was diagnosed as having glue ear. For that reason, she felt that he needed therapy to help him catch up on the development he had missed:

I suppose really he's got to develop his language really. I suppose he couldn't hear words before, like as a toddler.

In a similar way, Jacky and Gary made the decision for their little boy to start receiving therapy. His hearing levels appeared to vary quite a bit and they felt that this was affecting his progress:

He suffers a lot from catarrh . . . I think his hearing has got better 'til he gets a cold and then it's back to, you're back to square one again so I think it's to do with . . . the middle ear.

One mother chose to remain in the delayed therapy group, so that her little boy would qualify for the promised period of intensive help. However, when she spoke about her experience at the end of the project, Sally believed that her child's progress had been delayed for a year when they eventually came to receiving therapy at the end of the 12 months. He was only now starting to make real improvements when she felt he should have been completely better by this time:

I think he's missed an awful lot in a year . . . whereas last year because he hasn't seen anybody he's made less [*progress*] than what he probably could have made. **Sally**

While other things were happening in her child's life which she felt were positive in terms of encouraging his speech and language development, for example, starting nursery, in retrospect, Sally did question whether delaying speech and language therapy further was the right decision:

> I feel that he could have made a lot more progress and quicker if he had therapy sooner, which would have helped with his anger and tantrums and tears, and also with mixing with his peers.

A number of the parents interviewed who chose for their children to start receiving speech and language therapy felt that their child had benefited from treatment and that their decision to start therapy had been the right one:

> I had a bit more confidence that . . . I felt I could help and everybody was aware that there was a problem . . . so basically he's progressed well, which is good. **Fiona**

> I mean we'd tried hard with him . . . and I don't think that's good enough really . . . no, I don't think he would have been as good as what he is now. **Gary**

Some other parents had seen far less progress in their children and were far more uncertain about the effects of therapy. Hayley did not regret having decided to change options but had expected that greater progress would have been made. This left her feeling downhearted and wondering if she was to blame:

> It's not too bad but sometimes I feel like I've tried and is it me letting her down?

Changes in the opinions of the parents over the 12 months

Sometimes the parents' opinions changed over the course of the 12 months and they did feel differently looking back over the child's development. Carol, who agreed to delay therapy for her son, expressed the view that while she may have felt worried about waiting for treatment initially, this has proved successful for her and her child. She was pleased that therapy did not start immediately:

> I did think . . . we should be getting on with it now [*having therapy*] but then on the other hand it gave him a chance to sort of . . . come on on his own . . . he really turned a big corner and he done that all on his own. **Carol**

However, some parents stuck to their opinions throughout their time in the project and did not change their minds about how they felt. Sandra, who tried to reject early speech and language therapy involvement, became unhappy with attending therapy sessions for her son and after a short attendance asked for therapy to be terminated, wishing no further contact:

> It was making me feel lower as well because I felt as if they weren't really, nothing, nobody was really helping him like in a very positive way and it seemed a bit endless.

Other parents felt glad all the way through that their child had received therapy:

> I was pleased, it's been good . . . I'm glad that we went definitely. **Patricia**

From the accounts of the parents it is possible to see a number of factors at work which influenced the parents' preference for accepting early treatment or agreeing to delay it. These are summarized in Box 4.7.

BOX 4.7 FACTORS INFLUENCING THE PARENTS' PREFERENCE FOR IMMEDIATE OR DELAYED THERAPY

The parents preferred the immediate therapy or to change option when:

- they felt that there was an urgency for progress to be made
- they had difficulty in coping with the child's communication difficulties
- they felt that the rate of improvement was insufficient
- they were anxious about the child's ability to cope with the demands of school
- the child had either a history of or was still experiencing hearing loss.

The parents preferred delayed therapy when:

- they were satisfied with the progress being made by the child
- they were less concerned about the child's difficulty so that delaying therapy seemed natural
- they were curious to see how the child would develop if left to him/herself
- family circumstances made regular attendance at speech and language therapy difficult.

Considering the options

Following on from the assessment by the speech and language therapist, their accounts show that some of the parents preferred to receive therapy immediately, while others preferred to wait and see what happened to their children's speech and language development. As well as finding out what the parents thought of the options, an important part of the project was to explore the effects of immediate and delayed therapy on the children themselves. In Chapter 7, the progress the children made in the two treatment options in the course of the project will be presented and explored. Meanwhile, the next chapter will focus on how the parents whose children received immediate treatment felt about the process of therapy and the issues this process raised for them.

Summary of the chapter

- Following assessment, the speech and language therapist would normally discuss with parents what options existed for therapy and a way forward would be decided upon, which might include the child being placed on review or receiving some form of treatment immediately.
- The children of the parents who were interviewed were part of a research project. They were allocated either to immediate therapy or to delayed therapy.
- For some of the parents, having immediate therapy was acceptable. These parents were eager for progress to be made, had difficulty in coping with the child's communication difficulties and were anxious about the child's ability to cope with the demands of school. They also had concerns because their child had either a history of or was still experiencing conductive hearing loss.
- For other parents, delaying therapy was the preferred option. These parents felt the child was making progress, were less concerned about the difficulty and were curious to see how the child would develop on his/her own. Their family circumstances also made regular attendance at speech and language therapy difficult.

CHAPTER 5

The process of therapy

In Chapter 4, the focus was on the therapy options - immediate therapy and delayed therapy - and the responses of the parents to them. In the interviews the parents of children who had received treatment had the chance to talk about what therapy had been like for them. This chapter will explore in detail how these parents viewed the therapy their children received. They highlighted a number of issues connected with the process of therapy, which are shown in Box 5.1.

Box 5.1 ISSUES CONNECTED WITH THE THERAPY PROCESS DESCRIBED BY THE PARENTS

The organization of therapy.

Roles and responsibilities in therapy.

Emotional responses to the therapy process.

How the parents' views of therapy changed.

The organization of therapy

In the interviews, the parents made comments on a number of aspects of the organization of therapy. These included the flexibility and length of appointments, the frequency of the therapy sessions and the activities undertaken as part of the children's therapy.

The therapy appointments

The parents appeared to appreciate the flexibility of appointment times that were offered to them, especially where they were balancing bringing their children to the clinic with work and other commitments. For the majority of the parents, getting to the sessions did not pose any problems either, because the local clinic was close by:

> It's worked out OK for me because . . . it always fitted in with my work . . . and it's close by, only down the road, so it's quite easy for me to get to. So there hasn't been any problems with the practicalities of going. **Caroline**

> But it's no problem because I can more or less choose my own appointment times within reason, you know, out comes the book and . . . I've got my car so, it's no problem at all, no problem. **Patricia**

> There hasn't been too much of a problem with the practicalities. It was quite local 'cos we've gone to the health centre . . . it's only a 15 minute walk . . . the time was arranged to suit me. **Isabel**

The parents also appreciated being able to bring their other children to the clinic where necessary. Amy mentioned that she had been able to find babysitters for her younger child during her son's therapy sessions. She was pleased, however, that if this had not been possible, she would have been able to bring her other child along to the sessions as well:

> I mean I'm lucky enough I got a lot of people who could have her and also you can bring them with you, can't you?

Another parent appreciated the fact that her child was seen by the speech and language therapist in the nursery he was attending. This was very convenient for her and made additional clinic visits unnecessary, where she would have needed to bring her son's baby brother as well.

In the case of the children whose parents were interviewed, therapy sessions usually lasted about an hour. On the whole, the parents felt that the length of the appointments was about right. The parents were concerned that the appointments did not become too demanding, particularly when the child's concentration span was limited, as Monica's statement shows:

> I think it's enough, it is long enough, 'cos they sort of start getting fidgety but, yeah what they do in an hour is really good.

However the parents sometimes experienced other difficulties with the length of the therapy appointments. Fiona felt that there had not been sufficient time for discussion between her and the therapist at the end of the session, where she could talk to the therapist about the activities she would be carrying out with her son at home:

When I was saying that I would have liked more information for myself and more time to discuss how to do things with him . . . it would have been too long to have any more time after that session because it would have then probably, he would have got frustrated after that time.

The frequency of the therapy sessions

One of the aspects of the therapy process discussed by the parents which they most often found unsatisfactory was the frequency of the therapy appointments. A number of the parents had expected that therapy sessions would take place more frequently. Patricia had attended speech and language therapy for her two older sons and imagined that therapy appointments would take place as frequently for her third son as they did for the first two. This did not prove to be the case, as the sessions initially took place monthly followed by a gap of several months:

> I could remember my other boys were going quite regularly for quite a while whereas he [*her third son*] hasn't had very many visits at all.

Other parents who had had no previous experience of speech and language therapy also thought that the therapy sessions had not taken place often enough:

> I wish it had been a bit more often . . . 'cos it was once a fortnight, sometimes once every three weeks, even longer sometimes and I think it should be about once a week. **Amy**

Gary's little boy had been seen by the speech and language therapist about once a month and he was keen for him to be seen more often:

> If they turned round and said speech therapy will be every evening we'd be relieved and somehow we'd get him up there every evening.

Dorothy's son was seen even less frequently, with intervals of about three or four months between visits. For her, a monthly appointment would have been better as there would have been greater continuity in the therapy process:

> I mean she [*the therapist*] was asking me what I thought about his speech and that lot and obviously I was telling her when I thought it had improved . . . but I think it would have been better if she could have heard it on a monthly basis herself . . . and she could have made her own first hand assessment of him as each month went by.

However, one mother explained that during the time her little girl was being seen for therapy she became worried that other developmental difficulties were present and she wanted to seek another opinion. She reported that the amount of therapy her little girl was receiving was actually increased in response to the worries she expressed to the speech and language therapist:

> I felt very panicked at one point and sought other advice as well and at that point the therapist actually increased her sessions, the frequency of them, I think because she could sense that I was feeling a little bit more anxious. **Isabel**

The therapy activities

In the interviews, some of the parents spoke positively about the therapy activities which had taken place as part of their child's treatment, reporting that the activities had been enjoyed by both their child and by themselves:

> I think she took to it well. I don't think I could say there was anything wrong with it. **Selina**

> He enjoyed it and used to cooperate and he used to look forward to going. **Patricia**

> It's a good laugh, some of the games, especially the ones where he had to be the person that was in charge of the game . . . he'd enjoy that. **Gary**

Some of the parents whose children received therapy explained what the focus of the treatment sessions had been and why. Patricia's son had difficulties making himself understood. He also had some difficulties with understanding what was said to him and this was worked on in therapy:

> He was also the more, the understanding of words and how to put words together . . . for instance if somebody was stood next to something or he was behind the chair, he was confused with all that as well . . . so we used to concentrate more on games like that which we'd have little families at the table and I used to say, 'Can you put the rabbit under the table?' so he really had to listen and concentrate.

Hayley's daughter was speaking very little at the time she was receiving therapy. She described how therapy focused on improving her little girl's ability to concentrate, which she felt was holding back her learning of language:

> But I think what they concentrate on more with her is concentration than it is speech . . . she does speak to you and if I say words slowly with her she can actually put it all into a sentence . . . and she'll do that a couple of times and then

she'll lose interest and wanders off again but that's what I say, it is the concentration why there is a lack of speech.

However, for a few other parents the focus of the therapy activities became a difficult issue and affected the way they viewed the entire therapy process, as Caroline's, Sandra's and Dorothy's accounts in Box 5.2 reveal.

Box 5.2

Caroline, Sandra and Dorothy brought their children to speech and language therapy with strong expectations about what it would be like. All three of their children were experiencing problems with putting words together and with producing speech sounds. These mothers all imagined that the therapist would be concentrating on correcting the actual sounds that their children were making. Instead it focused on building up their children's vocabulary and encouraging them to put words together. The individual therapists working with these three children chose to concentrate on language development, rather than on the children's speech as their mothers had expected. They all became disillusioned with therapy when it did not appear to be tackling what they thought it would (or should). These parents could not recall having discussed with the therapist or having had an explanation about why language was being treated rather than speech. In fact, all three parents gained a similar impression that their child was not actually being 'treated' but merely re-assessed on each visit. This seemed to contribute especially to their disappointment with the service, as they felt that nothing specific was being worked on and they were being given little or no new advice. Their stories show a similar pattern:

> Really the learning he's done I sort of feel he's just done it 'cos he's done it, not because he went to speech therapy. It's just all happened in . . . the year. 'Cos I didn't have any set things that I was supposed to be doing with him. **Caroline**

> It [*therapy*] dragged on a bit and I stopped going. I told her [*the therapist*] I didn't want to go anymore 'cos I really felt as if it wasn't going anywhere . . . just felt as if it was a waste of time . . . I mean the boys had fun but didn't feel as if anything was being gained from it. **Sandra**

> Well, really it was what I was doing anyway, it's like playing games with him and getting him to say like the things you were playing with . . . it's what you do with your kids anyway . . . to be honest with you, I went away

> thinking what a waste of time . . . you go up there. His speech has improved a little bit but not a lot, and you're going away, doing exactly what you're doing the months prior to that, then you go back again and you're coming home, it's just going round in a circle. **Dorothy**

These parents were among the very few who expressed strong dissatisfaction with the process of therapy and thought the treatment had been of little practical value. Sandra had doubts about the therapy process all the way along but Caroline and Dorothy were happy for their children to start receiving therapy to begin with. When they had tried it, however, they were dissatisfied with what happened, unconvinced of the usefulness of the therapy and were reluctant to continue with it.

The accounts of the parents show it was possible for them to be satisfied with some aspects of the organization of therapy but to remain unhappy about others, particularly the amount of therapy they received. However, in the interviews, particularly those with Caroline, Sandra and Dorothy, it appeared vital that the parents could understand and accept the therapy activities done with their child. Where they could see no reasons for what was happening and did not perceive the activities as beneficial, real involvement of the parents in the therapy process did not seem to be possible.

Roles and responsibilities in therapy

When the parents spoke about the therapy they experienced, many of them mentioned that before attending speech and language therapy for the first time they had expected to take some part in the treatment process. Several of the parents had a fully-formed idea of what their own role was likely to be and how they and the therapist should be working together in partnership. These parents took it for granted that they would be 'doing therapy' with their children in between therapy sessions:

> **Interviewer:** What would you see it to be the speech and language therapist's job to do?
> **Sally:** To give me suggestions on how I could help him myself at home . . . I mean new ideas . . . and specific areas to work on . . . also to work alongside whatever the speech therapist is doing so that we're working together rather than me trying to do something and her trying to do something else.

> I mean I think their [*speech and language therapists'*] job as well is to like teach the parents, educate the parents as well because obviously you're with them most of the time. I think it's up to the parents to do as much really, I think. **Amy**

I think it's the speech therapist's job to help parents with the children to explain what they want them to do at home. **Hayley**

At the end of the day it's more of a two-way thing, it's more for us to do what we have to do to help him along and you're [*the therapist*] to advise on how we should go about doing it . . . it's as much our responsibility as it is for you to advise, it's more our responsibility to do the tasks. **Gary**

The parents who had had previous contact with speech and language therapy for other children had learnt from their earlier experiences that they would be involved in the therapy process:

'I know they . . . have these sessions where the kid's got sort of on a one-to-one basis . . . but it still does come down to what happens at home doesn't it? **Bernadette**

I assume as well that she's [*the therapist*] there for me as well . . . so I can help him when we're out of speech therapy . . . at home. **Patricia**

Other parents did not mention that they saw themselves as partners with the speech and language therapist in the process of therapy. However, it was clear from their comments that they were still actively following the therapist's advice and trying out activities with their child:

I used to say, 'I don't understand what you're saying.' The speech therapist used to say to me, 'Well, don't say that, just repeat the sentence,' and the bits that I get wrong my daughter'll pick me up on and that would encourage her to say the word properly. **Selina**

She [*the therapist*] also said like try and add more words . . . and when he says it wrong just to say it back how it should be. **Kate**

A couple of months ago it was *in*, *on* and *under* which she was having difficulty with. So if I'm at home now and there's teddy on the settee I say, 'Put teddy under the cushion', 'on the cushion' . . . I'd try and sort of make it playtime. **Monica**

All of these parents were involved in the therapy process, working with their children at home, following general advice given them by the speech and language therapist and doing specific activities. Yet it emerged from the accounts of the parents that even where they were carrying out therapy at home with their child, they still saw the therapist's role as crucial. The reasons for this were:

- The parents saw the speech and language therapist as the one who understood where the problems lay and then decided which areas needed to be worked on.
- The speech and language therapist was also thought of by parents as somebody who could provide ideas about how particular areas of difficulty could be worked on, in the form of advice or activities.

When they talked about their expectations of the therapy process in the interviews, it became clear that some of the parents had anticipated that the therapist would also provide the bulk of the therapy needed by the child in one-to-one sessions:

> I imagined it was going to be a bit more involved than it was . . . I guess a bit more one-to-one work with him with the problems rather than just assessing and telling me, give me an idea of how to deal with it and then going home with it. I guess I presumed there'd be a bit more . . . dealing with the particular areas that he couldn't, wasn't doing very well . . . I thought there was going to be more. **Fiona**

While the parents had expected to have a role in therapy, they did not think that this should mean being left to 'get on with it'. Fiona said that she had expected more to be done in the clinic. Instead she was faced with carrying out most of the work herself with less support than she had hoped for. She explained how she had tried to make the best of the situation:

> Take it on board, go home and do the best you can. As it happened, because he has improved and he's coped with it then to me, that's fine but if he hadn't improved I guess I would have gone back, thinking, you know, this isn't enough, please help more and do something more.

A number of the parents were surprised when they were expected to play such a large part in treatment. Their most common complaint was that there was not enough time set aside when they could talk to the therapist about the activities and games they should be trying out at home and write down the therapist's suggestions. A number of mothers mentioned the difficulties they experienced when trying to take notice of what was going on in the therapy session but having to look after other younger children at the same time. Jacky did not have anyone who could look after her younger son during therapy sessions so she had to take him with her. Sometimes he was so disruptive of the sessions that she had to take him out of the room altogether. This meant that she missed the chance to pick up on what the therapist was doing with her other son:

Yes, it's very difficult someone to look after my youngest one 'cos that's difficult but I can't be in the room, knowing everything that's happened.

Isabel's situation was the same as Jacky's:

I'm not very good at remembering things, also part of the sessions I have to say I mean with having a young baby with me as well, you know, my time, I was at times a little bit preoccupied with her if she wanted feeding or if she was a little bit restless. My attention wasn't completely full during the sessions.

Involving parents in speech and language therapy for pre-school children

It has become very common in speech and language therapy, particularly for young children, to closely involve their parents in the delivery of treatment. This has come about partly in recognition that parents are able to spend more time with their child than a therapist can. Moreover, the skills in speech, language and communication which therapy is seeking to develop are ones that are being repeatedly practised by children in their home environment. For that reason, many speech and language therapy services have aimed at the 'empowerment' of parents, that is, concentrating on transferring skills and knowledge to parents and carers, in order to equip them to deliver therapy at home. This has meant that nowadays the role of the speech and language therapists is a 'consultative' one, as they pass on more of the 'hands-on' work to parents. It was evident from the interviews that the majority of the parents imagined that they would be involved in the therapy process and that responsibility for what happened would be shared between them and the therapist. However, the extent to which they would be expected to become involved in therapy was not always spelled out to them in advance. This sometimes resulted in misunderstanding between the parents and therapists and in some disappointment for the parents.

The parents' accounts demonstrated that they were keen for their children to be seen by the speech and language therapist because they saw this as a way of getting help for them. However, some parents mentioned that they, too, were in need of help. Often they felt they wanted practical advice and ideas to cope with the speech and language difficulties but also mentioned that they needed support and reassurance for themselves. The parents who felt that these had been available were the ones for whom the therapy process was most satisfactory:

I didn't know how to deal with it, [*the difficulties*] you see. I found the speech therapy benefited me more at the time. She [*the therapist*] just explained to me how to deal with each problem, you know, how to help him. **Amy**

She [*the therapist*] was very good, she always explained . . . the reasons why, what she was doing . . . to get it across to me 'cos I used to come home and do things with him then and it was really good because some ideas that she was giving me I don't think I would ever have thought of . . . I think we both benefited from it. **Patricia**

Dorothy describes, however, what happened when parents did not feel they were being backed up by speech and language therapy. She felt that she was completely on her own in managing her son's difficulties:

It's not what the actual speech therapist does . . . but you sort of go up there . . . and you still come home and sort it out yourself like. Yeah, they put you on the right track . . . know what I mean but it's more at home than what it is up at speech therapy . . . you're just told to go home and continue the work at home.

While speech and language therapy services may be aiming to 'empower' parents, it appeared that the parents who took part in these interviews sometimes had different views about what was empowering for them. For a number of the parents, going ahead with their child's therapy enabled them to feel empowered, especially when they felt they received the advice and support necessary. As shown in the previous chapter, several parents felt empowered simply by being able to have their child's difficulties assessed followed by a waiting period to let the child develop with just help at home. For another parent, who did not agree with her son's referral to speech and language therapy in the first place, being empowered meant monitoring his development and referring him if the expected improvement did not take place. So for these parents, empowerment did not just signify therapists transferring skills to enable them to work with their children at home. They viewed it as something much wider, which took into account their wishes and circumstances and gave them help and support.

Emotional responses of the parents to the therapy process

In Chapters 1 and 2, the parents discussed the mixture of emotions they felt – guilt, concern and uncertainty – when their child's difficulties were first becoming apparent and when referral to speech and language therapy was being made. In the previous chapter, the parents' feelings about the therapy options and their emotional reactions were highlighted. In this chapter, the emotional responses of parents to the therapy process will now be considered. In the interviews, the parents commented on the ways in which the therapy process affected them at an emotional level. They experienced both positive and negative feelings in the course of the therapy process.

Positive feelings about the therapy process

It was clear from the interviews that for a number of the parents the therapy process had been a positive and reassuring experience. In previous sections of this chapter, the parents talked about the organization of therapy and the roles and responsibilities in the therapy process. The therapy process appeared to be positive for parents when:

- they agreed with therapy going ahead
- they felt that the amount of therapy sessions was reasonable. If they wanted more it was because they felt therapy was successfully helping their child
- they felt they had enough practical ideas to help the child at home
- they received support for themselves from the therapist.

Parents also gained in confidence during the therapy process when they could see that their child's difficulties were changing and improving, as these parents' statements illustrate:

Everything she's [*the therapist*] done with him has worked. I've been happy with it all. **Amy**

It helped me to help him really, to have more of the confidence to know that I was doing it right . . . all the while he's progressed. **Patricia**

Linda's and Jacky and Gary's little boys both started their treatment after six months of waiting. These parents spoke very positively about what has happened since the therapy process got underway:

He knows certain sounds and what they should sound like so it has done him a world of good, to be honest, yeah I'm pleased with it. **Linda**

We're absolutely convinced that without the therapy, there wouldn't have been improvement, absolutely. I'd put the house on it . . . I mean he's bound to improve a little bit with nursery and everything but there's just no way it would have been as significant as it has been. Very encouraging. **Gary**

A few parents commented also on how it was possible for them to feel worried about their children's development but not to be taken seriously by others around them. As Dorothy pointed out, having speech and language therapy confirmed that her child was experiencing difficulties which people might otherwise dismiss. She contrasts her situation with that of other mothers she has known:

You know, 'cos with some kids like . . . you're made to feel a bit neurotic about it, aren't you though, over-reacting like . . . I have had a couple of friends who've said they've been made to feel well they're just stupid mothers basically, there's nothing wrong with their kids' speech, when there have been as far as the parents have been concerned.

Negative feelings about the therapy process

For a number of parents, however, the process of therapy had inspired more negative reactions. These are displayed in Box 5.3.

Box 5.3 Negative feelings about the therapy process reported by the parents

Feeling worried.

Feeling inadequate as a parent.

Feeling stigmatized by the therapy process.

Feeling worried

For some of the parents who were dissatisfied with the treatment their child received, the therapy process came to be source of concern to them. Sandra explained how she felt the therapy process had had damaging effects on her, by making her question how she and her son had got on together in the past. Her son's speech and language had not been a matter for concern before and she had always been happy with the way they communicated with each other:

> It [*therapy*] did do damage in the sense of making me worry, because we'd always got on really well.

While she felt that her relationship with her son hadn't suffered as a result, she was unhappy because she felt that she had been forced to admit that he was experiencing difficulties. Like Sandra, Dorothy had been dissatisfied with therapy and did not feel that it had achieved anything. The therapy process raised much concern for her, particularly as she began to think of the future. Knowing that her child's problems were persisting, she questioned what could be done to help him:

> I can't see what difference it will make. Not if what I've had already is anything to go by. You know, you keep on doing the things at home with him and what

happens if his speech doesn't improve? I mean where does it go then? . . . I mean is there another step that . . . for children like him who are really slow in learning to speak or do we just keep on treading the mill.

Feeling inadequate

Hayley's little girl was allocated to delayed therapy but she chose for her to start receiving therapy after a wait of six months because the difficulties were not getting better. Hayley explained how during the therapy process she had felt patronized by the speech and language therapist they saw. She felt that the therapist did not show much understanding of her financial situation by expecting her to buy games for her daughter which she wasn't able to afford. Nor did she did feel that the therapist had been realistic about ways in which she could help her daughter. This left her feeling inadequate and very unsupported in the process of therapy:

> **Hayley:** I wish . . . they'd realize that not everybody can go out and buy these things for their kids and that there should be things that they can help you with more. I think she [*the therapist*] could give you a lot more advice and make you feel a lot better about yourself, 'cos it's your daughter that can't do it. Sometimes they speak to you as like well, you could do this, you could do that but you are doing it and sometimes you do blame yourself 'cos they don't give you the encouragement as well that you need when you're there.
> **Interviewer:** What would you have liked the speech therapist to have done?
> **Hayley:** Well, I would have liked her to have been more like, not a speech therapist, like a friend or someone who's there . . . I think to myself if you haven't got a lot of money, she should explain something like that to you to help her . . . she should be a bit more considerate of people that haven't got it, that can't do it.

Another mother whose child received treatment spoke of how she had felt inadequate in the course of therapy. She mentioned how she had been criticized by the speech and language therapist for emphasizing key words when she spoke to her son. But at the same time, she did not feel that the therapist was clearly indicating what she should be doing instead:

> But seeing that everything else was sort of vague and unstructured it seemed slightly odd that she [*the therapist*] was . . . specifically pinpointing the way that I reacted with him. So it didn't make me feel great, no. **Caroline**

Feeling stigmatized

For a number of the parents, feelings of stigma came about during the process of therapy. Marianne expressed the sense of loneliness she felt when her little boy had difficulties with learning to talk. When they attended the speech and language therapy sessions at the clinic she got the feeling that everybody was staring at her and her son. She knew that this was not the case but the experience of coming along to the therapy sessions was not an easy one for her.

Gary was one of the three fathers who were interviewed. He felt some embarrassment at the reactions of other children to his son's speech difficulties, as this statement shows:

> It was awful in the early stages . . . he would be blabbering about something, nobody would understand a word he was saying and his friend who's only a couple of months older than him turned round and said, 'What's he saying? Mummy, what's he saying?' and it was just awful . . . and another one of his friends said, 'He can't talk properly.'

Gary also felt slightly uncomfortable about the fact that his son was attending speech and language therapy:

> I mean it's not the sort of thing you blab on to people, 'Oh yeah, our son's going to speech therapy', shout it from the rooftops. I mean you do tend to keep that a little bit sort of quiet, you don't really want people to, you don't drum it into people that he's got a problem with his speech.

In a similar way, Selina's account in Box 5.4 illustrates the stigmatizing attitudes she came up against when her daughter experienced speech and language difficulties and attended therapy.

Box 5.4

Selina recounted incidents where she felt her little girl's speech and language difficulties had provoked discrimination from others. This caused her considerable distress:

> That used to upset me because it was like innocent little things like people used to say, 'Hello what's your name?' And she wouldn't answer . . . I just used to go, 'Oh she don't really talk a lot at the moment' and you could see the expression on their face and think, 'Yeah . . . she should be old enough to do that by now.' That was hard. It's just other people make you feel . . . like you felt that there's, like there's something wrong 'cos she ain't doing it like everybody else has.

Selina received speech and language therapy herself when she was a schoolgirl and for that reason, regarded speech and language therapy as 'not something to be frightened of'. She was happy for her daughter to be referred to speech and language therapy when her language development was delayed. However, even in her own family, she felt that no one understood this and that many of them still thought that something must be really wrong with a child for therapy to be necessary. She related how surprised family members were when they found out her daughter had been attending speech and language therapy:

> And a lot of people I think especially at family get-togethers they say, 'Oh she's getting on well'. 'Yeah, that's speech therapy' and they look at you and say, 'Well, what is she having speech therapy for? I didn't realize she could be that bad.'

For some of the parents who took part in the interviews, however, feelings of stigma arising from contact with speech and language therapy did not come about. They willingly accepted the need to go through the process of therapy with their children. They regarded this as part and parcel of being a parent, as these statements reveal:

> As far as I'm concerned whatever problem he comes across, we can, you know, do the best we can to, I mean he is who he is. **Fiona**

> I just think at the end of the day you're there to help the child, you're not there for you. **Hayley**

> It's like taking them to the doctor's or dentist really isn't it, you don't feel stigmatized by 'cos they got to go to the doctor's or the dentist. **Dorothy**

Bernadette and Ross had experienced how other parents regarded having speech and language therapy or help from other child health professionals as stigmatizing:

> It is I think some parents put it as a social downfall that it's either your kid's thick or it's our problem the child's suffering with a problem . . . you can't put this mark on people because they've been to speech therapy, they've got a massive problem . . . you ought to have seen the attitude we used to get when our daughter used to see a psychologist. People used to literally, you'd see them jump out of their skin. **Bernadette**

Ross explained that he has qualms about accepting professional help for himself and is suspicious of what some services can offer him. However, when it comes to his children, he wants to do all he can for them:

I think my attitude perhaps, personally I'm not prejudiced but the thought of me seeing a psychologist or a therapist, because you don't do that sort of thing but when it's the children, as far as I'm concerned anything like that goes out the window if it's going to help them.

Thus, Bernadette and Ross were determined to resist any feelings of stigma when their youngest child saw the speech and language therapist.

How the parents' views of therapy changed

The parents' descriptions of the emotional aspects of receiving speech and language therapy for their children reveal that therapy may provide reassurance but may also be a troubling process for them to deal with. The parents' accounts also show how it was possible for their feelings about the therapy process to change in the course of 12 months. For several parents, initial feelings of concern were replaced with confidence in the therapy process. For a few other parents, hopeful expectations of the therapy process ended in disappointment.

When looking across the accounts of the parents, it is possible to see how the parents had different anxieties and aims at different points in the course of the therapy process. Initially, when the parents were experiencing their first contact with speech and language therapy, their concerns and hopes were focused on entering the system and finding out what it could offer them and their child. At this point, perhaps, the expectations of the parents were at their strongest. In the interviews, Caroline, Sandra and Dorothy reported how their preconceptions came face-to-face with the reality of the speech and language therapy provision available. This early experience went on to affect their later attitudes toward therapy and what they felt it had (and had not) achieved with their children.

At this stage in the process also, the fear of the unknown was uppermost in the minds of the parents, as speech and language therapy represented uncharted territory for many of them. During this phase, it was usual for the parents to feel rather powerless and certainly less powerful than the therapist. The parents were likely to see the therapist as the expert making the decision about whether therapy was necessary. However, where the parents felt that during their early contact with the service, their child's problems had been clearly identified and explained by the therapist and they felt that they could relate to the therapist, their confidence in the therapy process began to grow. Thus, the experience of their initial encounters with speech and language therapy appeared to be extremely important in determining how the parents coped with the rest of the therapy process.

When they talked about their experience of the therapy process once actual treatment was underway, the parents expressed less fear and uncertainty than in the previous phase. Most of them felt that 'something was being done' for their child, which helped to reduce their worries. Some of the parents had been concerned that what they were trying to do to help their child might not have been the right thing and during this phase their fears were often put aside. Thus, as the parents became more familiar with speech and language therapy, for many of them the uncertainty of the previous phase was replaced with assurance. This phase involved establishing the roles of the therapist and parent and routines for therapy both in clinic and at home. Throughout this time also, the parents were judging how their children were responding to the therapy being received and whether the children were making progress with it.

Some of the parents easily settled into a pattern of attendance at the clinic and carrying out treatment at home. The majority of the parents whose children received therapy saw themselves as having a definite role in the therapy process, in partnership with the therapist. For other parents, however, things did not go so smoothly. Several parents found that their ideas regarding what treatment should involve, which they had held before their contact with speech and language therapy, clashed with the actual therapy process. This, in turn, affected how they looked upon the therapy process and interfered with their involvement. Thus when these parents felt that the help they needed was not being made available or that the therapy was not focusing on the areas they considered important, their enthusiasm for therapy dwindled.

This and the previous chapter have considered the responses of parents to therapy. In the next chapter the focus will be on how the parents responded to the research process and being involved in a speech and language therapy project.

Summary of the chapter

- In the interviews, the parents of the children who had received treatment mentioned a number of issues connected with the therapy process. These included the organization of therapy, roles and responsibilities in therapy, their emotional responses to the therapy process and how these changed in the course of therapy.
- With regard to the way in which therapy was organized, the parents generally expressed positive views about the flexibility and length of the appointments they and their children were offered.
- The frequency of the therapy sessions, however, was a matter of some concern to a number of the parents. Some of the children were seen every

two weeks, for others their sessions took place on a monthly basis. It seemed that if weekly therapy had been available, many of the parents would have preferred this.

- When they talked about the activities which had taken place as part of therapy, some of the parents reported that the activities had been enjoyable for their child and for themselves. A few other parents were disappointed because they did not feel that the therapy activities were being targeted at the right areas of difficulty experienced by their child.
- Many of the parents had expected that they would work together with the speech and language therapist to improve their child's difficulties.
- However, some of the parents imagined their child would receive more direct help from the therapist. Others did not feel that they were given the help and support they needed to carry out therapy with their child at home.
- Speech and language therapists are aiming to transfer skills and knowledge to parents for them to undertake therapy with their children. However, the parents expressed slightly different ideas about what would help them best.
- The parents expressed positive and negative feelings about the therapy process in which they were involved. Many of the parents felt that the therapy process had caused them to feel worried, inadequate as a parent and stigmatized.
- The parents' emotions underwent some changes in the course of the therapy process. For some parents, their early fears were set aside, they involved themselves in the process and they found therapy reassuring. For some others, their expectations of the therapy process were not met at an early stage and they became disillusioned by it.

CHAPTER 6

Responding to research

The involvement of the parents and their children in research

In the course of the interviews the parents expressed their views on their children's difficulties, referral to speech and language therapy, the therapy options to which their children had been allocated and the process of therapy. As well as talking about these issues, the parents often described in the interviews how they felt about being involved in a research project and their opinions about research itself. Being involved in a research project may or may not mean that the parents' experiences were similar to those of other parents whose children are attending speech and language therapy in normal service settings. However, a lot of research is being carried out in the UK. For that reason, it is useful to know how the parents felt about participating in research. This chapter will look more closely at a range of topics connected with the subject of research which were highlighted by the parents (shown in Box 6.1).

BOX 6.1 TOPICS ON THE SUBJECT OF RESEARCH EXPRESSED BY THE PARENTS

The parents explained what participation in the research meant to them.

The parents discussed their motivation to take part in the research project.

The parents described what they understood about the research project.

The meaning of participation in the research to the parents

Because they were all willing to participate in the project, the parents demonstrated their support for research into children's development. While they had given consent for their children to become involved in the research, it also became clear that participating in the project had a meaning for the parents themselves. This meaning was expressed by the parents in either positive or negative terms. It was influenced by where the parents felt they stood in relation to society.

On the positive side, a number of parents saw their participation in the project as a way of giving something back to society which had provided help for their child in the first place:

> I'm pleased that we did it . . . you feel as though you're helping giving something back . . . as well as still having treatment which she would have had anyway. **Emma**

> I felt very positive about being part of a research programme . . . it can't always be somebody else that does it for you. There are times when you, you know, you have to be prepared to actually sort of do it yourself. **Isabel**

On the negative side, one mother expressed the view that society was demanding a lot of a parent by asking them to give consent for their child to participate in this type of research, where therapy for the child might end up being delayed:

> I mean we were asking for help for our child with his speech and language development and weren't particularly interested in being moved into a research group. **Fiona**

Sandra complained that the research was only necessary because health care professionals had taken control of children's normal development and interfered unnecessarily. This did mean, however, that she was keen to take part in the research because it provided a chance to look at children's progress in an objective way and limit the over-involvement of professionals:

> I was quite interested in doing the research because I had my doubts myself [*about the need for speech and language therapy*].

The parents' ideas about the meaning of taking part in the research were also affected by how they felt society perceived them. Several parents explained how they often felt judged when speech and language difficulties arose in their child, which they believed they might have caused by their own behaviour or handling of the child. Where the parents were feeling under-confident about their own skills and ability to deal with their child's difficulty, this in turn affected how the immediate therapy and delayed therapy groups of the project were perceived. One mother who had questioned whether she could be to blame for her little boy's difficulties expressed the urgency she felt to sort out the problems. Her son was allocated to delayed therapy but made good progress over the 12 months. She felt that being in the delayed therapy group could have increased this sense of urgency, especially if the difficulties did not seem to be getting better:

> I'd felt as though perhaps there was anything else we could do, you know, to help him a lot more . . . I would have been a bit dismayed really. **Carol**

Another mother stated that if her son had been allocated to the delayed therapy group, she would have been expected to deal with his problems without much support. However, as a single parent she would, in all likelihood, be scapegoated for the wider ills of society if her child went on to fail at school:

> I felt that like if your kid's got a problem it's because you're a single parent. **Dorothy**

Several other parents felt that getting help for their child's difficulty was a priority over helping with the research because that was what was expected of them as parents. The parents who opted for their children to start receiving treatment took the view that they had done what they needed to do as parents to give their child a fair opportunity of catching up on devel-opment they had missed:

> I couldn't justify saying, 'OK, we'll go along with this research group and wait for a year,' because he needed help then. **Fiona**

Thus the interviews revealed that taking part in a research project prompted the parents to question their own standing in relation to the rest of society and how they were regarded by society, particularly in their role as parents. While many of the parents viewed participation in the research as positive, others felt resentful and as if they were being judged.

The parents' reasons for taking part in the research

When parents made their decision to participate in the research project, it appeared that a number of different motives influenced their thinking.

Certainly, the parents' explanations showed that they were taking both the interests of their own child and the interests of others into account. Thinking about the advantages of participating in the research for themselves, some of the parents expressed the view that by taking part in the research they would be getting the best treatment for their child. They felt that they would be better looked after by being in a research project. For this reason, Ross was prepared for his son to be included in the project:

> It was fine, if he's going to benefit from being part of the project, well fine.

He also felt that the allocation to the immediate therapy group or to the delayed therapy group would take their circumstances into account and favour them:

> If she'd [*the therapist*] seen something . . . and thought . . . this is something really serious well then he wouldn't have been put on that sort of waiting group.

The parents also expressed concern that their actions would help others, demonstrating that they wanted to do not only what was best for their own child but also what was best for the children who would follow later. So they viewed taking part in the research positively, as a way of gaining knowledge for the benefit of future children:

> I think everything needs to be researched especially for children . . . it could be the next year, the next child or the next one, they might need help exactly the same as her but they could be the same, they might not need speech therapy but they might need a few pointers in the right direction. **Hayley**

> I think it's necessary to have this project. I think if we don't have it then we're not going to know. **Emma**

A number of parents expressed their hope that their own experience could be turned into better provision for others:

> I mean that's why I agreed to go on this 'cos I thought maybe in future . . . there might be a different way of going around doing it. **Dorothy**

However, less positively, some parents viewed participation in the research as doing what was expected of them and some felt that this was too much. One mother explained that she had no objections to giving information abut her son's difficulties and his being assessed but did not want to risk his progress by having to wait for therapy:

I don't mind answering the questions . . . and assessing him . . . but it's just the fact
. . . I wish it was . . . therapy a lot more [*wish more therapy had been available*].
Jacky

All of the parents who were interviewed, however, whether they viewed the research positively or not, wanted to receive information about the findings and showed their ongoing interest in the research to which they had personally contributed.

The parents' understanding of the research project

When they talked about their participation in the research, the parents also described their understanding of the project a year after they had agreed to take part. At their initial appointment with the speech and language therapist, all the parents were given an explanation and written information about the project, before they consented to take part. In the interviews 12 months later, some of the parents were able to remember the aims of the research, although there was a range of understanding both of what the project was attempting to find out and how it was organized.

Some parents felt that there was a need for the project because they too wondered whether their child would get better without any help and if attending speech and language therapy earlier really was better. Patricia, whose three sons all received speech and language therapy, expressed this uncertainty:

I mean I'm assuming that speech therapy has helped all my children but would they have got there on their own?

She proposed a rather drastic way of carrying out the research, but one that comes close to the actual design of the project – the only difference being that instead of dividing individual children in half the whole sample of children are divided up and assigned to different groups and then compared:

It would be interesting if you could cut them in half . . . let them have therapy and just leave them alone and see what comes.

Other parents, however, were unable to view the project as an attempt to find out if children needed therapy because they already felt that therapy was needed for the difficulties. Some parents considered it wrong and unethical to withhold a treatment, even where its value was not proven, as was the case for speech and language therapy for pre-school children at the time of the research:

> I was told yes, he had a problem . . . and I think now, well, I've got to wait . . . to get any help. **Linda**

Perhaps because of this, a few parents saw the research as an opportunity for the researchers to find out how to 'do therapy' rather than to find out if it had any impact on the difficulties. Other parents saw the project as a way of saving money, as only half the children received immediate treatment:

> It was a case of if his name came out of the box . . . then he was lucky enough to go on it . . . which I think is wrong . . . but then I suppose it's all the cutbacks. **Dorothy**

These statements demonstrate the range of beliefs and assumptions about the research which existed among the parents who agreed to take part.

It is likely that the parents' attitudes to this project were dependent upon a number of factors such as:

* their individual personality and how they responded to the explanation of the research given them
* the accuracy of the information about the project they received from the speech and language therapist in the beginning
* how they made sense of the information at that point and over the period of their involvement in the project
* their accuracy in recalling the information after 12 months.

However, a year after they had agreed to participate, it became clear in the interviews that the parents welcomed the chance to discuss the project again and to receive an explanation of its purposes. Their accounts also showed that when the parents had ongoing access to information about the aims and organization of the project and chance to discuss them, they tended to be more positive about their participation.

Exploring the views of people who take part in research

The interviews with the parents whose children took part in this project show exactly how the parents reflected on what the research meant for them, their reasons for being involved and how they understood the research. Other projects have shown that these parents are not alone in the way they gave such issues a lot of consideration. Clearly, when people give consent to take part in projects their opinions about the meaning, purpose and aims of the research are of importance, as these may affect how people cooperate in the research process. Today in the National Health Service there is a growing understanding of how necessary it is to explore how people who take part in research view that research.

The focus of this chapter has been on the parents' opinions of the research they took part in. In the next chapter, the views and feelings of the parents about their children's progress in the course of the project will be explored.

Summary of the chapter

- In the interviews, the parents discussed their views on their involvement in the research project and research in general.
- The parents explained what participation in the research meant to them. The meaning of their participation was influenced both by where they felt they stood in relation to society and how society perceived them in their role as parents.
- The parents discussed their motivation to take part in the research project. The reasons they gave for taking part showed that they took both the needs of their own children and other children into account.
- The parents described their understanding of the research project. Their accounts showed a range of ideas about the aims and organization of the project.
- When parents received adequate information about the project during the time of their involvement, they felt more positive about participation.
- In the National Health Service today there is a growing emphasis placed on understanding the views of people who take part in research about the research.

CHAPTER 7

Looking at the children's progress

The parents whose accounts are reported in this book were interviewed about a year after their contact with speech and language therapy had begun. Over the course of the 12 months, some of the parents had undergone therapy with their children and others had agreed to monitor their child's difficulties while therapy was delayed. The purpose of this chapter is to describe:

- how the parents and the children had coped with the difficulties over the year
- if, and in what way, the parents believed their children's difficulties had changed over the course of the year and what difficulties they felt still remained
- the parents' feelings about the point their child had reached
- what they expected would happen in the future
- the matters they revealed as being sources of continuing concern to them.

At the end of the chapter a review of recent research will show what is known about the course of early speech and language delays and the effects of speech and language therapy on them.

Coping with the difficulties

Over the course of the year, both the parents and the children themselves lived with the speech and language difficulties on a day-to-day basis. Some of the parents described the ongoing frustrations in dealing with their child's speech and language problems and the impact of the difficulties on the child and those around them. A number of parents commented on how they were finding it extremely hard just to know what their child wanted or was trying to tell them:

I'd be trying to say things with her and then finding it wasn't really what she wanted at all, it was nothing to do with it and then she'd get frustrated with me because I couldn't understand. We just couldn't really understand what she was saying. **Emma**

We'd have to try, it's like a guessing game, you'd try and say so many words and then go through them all until she sort of went 'Yeah' . . . eventually you'd get there but it just took a long time. **Selina**

Sometimes you just couldn't [*understand*] he would cry his eyes out . . . and then he would start shouting at you because he knew what he was trying to say. **Gary**

I used to feel upset quite a bit, like I mean sometimes even now she'll sort of try and have a conversation with you and it still comes out wrong and . . . I feel more sorry for her really 'cos she can't sort of say what she's done during the day. **Monica**

Several parents mentioned that their child was prone to having temper tantrums when they could not make themselves understood. Sally was worried about the effects this was having on her son's relationships with his friends:

I know what he's been like in the last year and because he gets so cross and so angry, not necessarily communicating with adults because adults learn to understand what he's saying but he's got so many little friends . . . but they get cross with him 'cos they tell him to speak properly.

Carol was also concerned about how her son's speech and language difficulties were affecting his behaviour and the way he interacted with other children:

He wouldn't communicate at all really because he'd go up to a child and take a toy off and that child would get upset and he'd bite or smack or do something like that because he could not communicate.

Other mothers mentioned how they got used to the way their child talked and were then expected to be his 'translator' by other people:

I think as a mother you just get to know what little sounds mean . . . even now, yeah, he's talking a lot but people always look at me and say, 'What did he say?' **Linda**

The majority of people would say 'What did he say?', but I was finding that I was speaking for him as well because he'd say, he'd ask a question and then I'd say it again for him. **Patricia**

Both mothers felt that this affected how their child felt about talking. Linda believes that her son has become aware that he can't be understood and that this has undermined his confidence:

I think he's probably getting aware that people aren't understanding him and I think this is what's knocked his, he's not a confident child and I think this is probably why.

Changes in the difficulties after a year

After a year, all the parents who were interviewed reported that they had seen changes come about in their child's difficulties. However, the amount of change the parents spoke of varied enormously and this determined how the parents viewed their child's outcome, as Box 7.1 demonstrates.

Box 7.1 How the parents viewed their child's outcome after 12 months

Some parents believed that their child's difficulties had resolved.

Some parents believed that their child was still experiencing some difficulties but that these were on the way to getting better.

Some parents believed that their child still had major difficulties.

A few of the parents felt that their child's difficulties had sorted themselves out over the course of the year. Bernadette and Ross's little boy had been referred for difficulties with his speech sounds and his therapy was delayed for a year. At the end of this time, both of his parents felt that he was doing well with his talking and did not require any therapy at all at this point:

It's nice to have, sort of believe his speech is sorted out now. **Ross**

He doesn't need much help now. He didn't have any trouble communicating when he went down the school for the afternoon. **Bernadette**

Andrea's son was referred to speech and language therapy because of the clarity of his speech and his therapy was also delayed. She spoke of the changes that had happened during the year's wait and was confident that he did not need therapy any more:

> I said to his Dad the other day that he probably talks better than a lot of the other ones now. He is just so, you know, grown-up with his talking, the things he comes out with, you know, and he's quite precise. He's come on in leaps and bounds. **Andrea**

Bernadette and Andrea mentioned that their children did sometimes have difficulties with making themselves understood and with particular sounds. They both felt that this was not a real problem and that their sons were coping very well:

> There may be a couple of little incidences . . . because if he can't say something to make, like even now sometimes there's some words that I don't understand, he will make you understand by going about it a different way. **Bernadette**

> It's only the 's' words that he still has a bit of a problem with but even that's getting better and he even sometimes he'll say a word and he'll say, 'I said that better that time, didn't I?' so even he knows, you know, when something's getting better. **Andrea**

A number of the parents felt that their child's difficulties were now on the way to being sorted out and were encouraged by the progress they had seen. Amy and Patricia, whose sons had both received therapy, felt that they had made big improvements:

> He's a lot better . . . he is much clearer . . . he don't seem to get quite so frustrated or anything. Like at playgroup, they just seem to understand him, so yeah he's doing quite well, I think. **Amy**

> He speaks a lot more clearly now than a lot of the other children . . . and his teacher can understand him, no problem, so I feel then that there's not really a problem, he's making, you know, he's getting on with it. **Patricia**

To begin with, Sandra was not convinced that her son had a problem which required him to be referred to speech and language therapy. She reported after 12 months that he had now started school and in terms of his talking was managing well:

> He's clear enough to cope and he's enjoying it . . . I mean he still obviously needs to carry on improving but he's obviously enjoying it and he's coping with it.

Fiona believed that her little boy's difficulties had got better during the year:

> I'm happy with the talking, there's no problem at all.

However, there were still aspects of his communication which needed to improve. Nevertheless she expected that he would make the progress in time:

> There's no problem with his vocabulary and his pronunciation is great . . . he's just lacking in understanding and socially . . . that is still a problem but I guess with time that will fall together . . . I'm just presuming that will, you know level itself out by the end of the year.

Similarly, Gary pointed out that his little boy was still lagging behind other children but the amount of progress he had made had been very pleasing:

> He's still not right, you know, he's still behind where some of his other friends are, still behind but I mean certainly . . . certainly it's more pleasant now and you can actually talk to him and understand him, he'll have a conversation with you . . . we feel that there's still a little bit to go, there's certainly more room for improvement . . . but the improvement has been there and it's been really exciting and encouraging.

While a number of the parents had been reassured by the progress their children had made and were confident that the difficulties would be sorted out, other parents felt that their children were still experiencing serious problems. The following statements illustrate what these children were like and the sort of difficulties they still had, in the eyes of their parents, at the end of the year:

> I don't think he talks very well . . . I would like him to speak better. It worries me that he's still got the same problems now a year on. **Caroline**

> She does get frustrated when you have a conversation, she wants, she wants to say something and she doesn't know yet, she doesn't understand to wait then to speak. **Hayley**

> I mean he has and still has got quite a bad speech problem, you can't hold a proper conversation . . . you can't hold a conversation with him, about four words strung together you can just about understand. It is still very babyish I must admit. **Dorothy**

I think a lot of people still have a problem with trying to comprehend what it is that she's saying . . . she still gets frustrated if she's not understood immediately. **Isabel**

The parents' feelings about their child's progress

When they talked about their child's progress over the course of the 12 months and their outcome at that point, the parents described their feelings. These are set out in Box 7.2.

Box 7.2 HOW THE PARENTS FELT ABOUT THEIR CHILD'S OUTCOME

Happy with the outcome for their child.

Unhappy with the outcome for their child.

Unsure about the outcome for their child.

Feeling happy about the outcome

A number of the parents felt happy about their child's progress over the year and with the point they had reached in addressing the difficulties. Emma's little girl's speech and language therapy had been delayed for a year. When Emma was interviewed, her daughter's therapy had begun a few weeks earlier. Emma's statement reveals her satisfaction with her daughter's progress and what was being done for her at that time:

> She's a different child, she's really much better . . . she's not so frustrated . . . her speech is much better so from that respect she's doing really really well. There's times when she's still not there but I think she's benefited totally from having speech therapy.

Even where the child's difficulties were not completely sorted out, as with Emma's daughter, some of the parents were content that their child's speech and language appeared to be moving in the right direction. Linda's son started receiving treatment for his speech and language difficulties after his therapy had been delayed for six months. She felt that he had made huge improvements in the course of the whole 12 months:

> I mean compared to last year he's ten times better than he was last year.

Linda also felt that therapy had helped her son get to the point he had now reached:

> In his case I think therapy did help, yeah. Yes, definitely.

Although she appreciated that his therapy would need to continue, she was happy with the outcome for her child after a year and felt that he would continue to improve with the right help.

Feeling unhappy about the outcome

There were several parents, however, who were far less happy with the progress their child had made in the year. Caroline believed that her little boy had improved in the 12 months since their first contact with speech and language therapy. However, she felt that he was still experiencing significant problems and the therapy he had received had not made a difference to his outcome:

> I don't feel it's [*the therapy*] made a difference . . . because I don't feel he's really benefited from going to speech therapy . . . I think he's just progressed as he normally would.

Caroline was sceptical about receiving any more therapy at the clinic in the future as she did not think it would make any difference to her son:

> With the speech therapy that's available to me I wouldn't actually be bothered if she [*the therapist*] said she didn't need to see him any more because I can't really see the point in going.

Dorothy told a similar story to Caroline's. Improvement in her son's difficulties had come about slowly and appeared to have come to a stop altogether at the end of the year, as her comment shows:

> He has improved but it's been a slow process . . . at the moment he does seem to have come to a standstill.

Dorothy was critical of the therapy her son had received and questioned what any future therapy could do for him:

> I don't think it [*therapy*] makes much difference personally myself.

Feeling unsure about the outcome

Another parent, Patricia, felt that her son had made good progress over the course of the 12 months and that therapy had benefited him. However, she still felt uncertain about the outcome for her child, particularly as his hearing levels carried on fluctuating. Because the presence of long-term hearing loss had not been established beyond doubt, his speech and language therapy had been put on hold. As Patricia herself described, this situation was a difficult one for her and her son where they were waiting to see what would happen:

> Ideally I need to get his ears sorted out and then go back and see her [*the therapist*] and get it all, nice and tidy so that we know . . . it's sort of in limbo.

She felt that if his hearing problems had been dealt with he could have received more therapy:

> I feel he's progressed but the whole thing in a way . . . has been a bit drawn out . . . I mean if his last test [*for hearing*] had not been very clever again . . . he'd have probably had his grommets [*a tube inserted surgically into the eardrum to ventilate the middle ear*] in by now and that side of it . . . would have been put right so . . . so maybe he would have seen the speech therapist more, more frequently then.

As well as speaking about the changes that had come about in their child's difficulties and describing their feelings about the point their child had reached, the parents also talked about their hopes and expectations for the future.

The parents' expectations for the future

Although all of the children whose parents were interviewed had improved in the course of the year, many were still experiencing some difficulties after this time. Because of the progress they had seen, the parents remained optimistic about the prospects for the child. However, they were also realistic about how much effort and time might still be necessary before their child could cope with all the demands made of them in nursery and at school:

> I mean it's not going to happen overnight, it's going to take time, and I would really like to see him improve before he goes to school . . . I think it's going to be very very difficult. **Sally**

> I think in general she's coming on, she's getting better. I think there's still a little way to go. Again you can see how frustrated she was getting trying to tell me something . . . I think that needs to be worked perhaps. **Emma**

> Well, I mean I'm happy with the talking, there's no problem at all. I'm waiting for his understanding to catch up and just, um . . . so he can socially fit in, so when he goes to school that he's going to be able to progress alright. **Fiona**

I think he will improve, I . . . believe now that he will actually be where he should be. I don't think he's there yet but I think the more encouragement and tuition that he will hopefully before he goes to school, he'll be where he should be at that age. **Gary**

While the parents were keen that their child's speech and language development should be moving on, many of them did not have a definite idea of what they were aiming for. As one parent expressed her idea of what she wanted for her child:

Normal, don't know what normal is . . . but normal. **Marianne**

Even where the children had been receiving regular speech and language therapy, the parents often did not recall any discussion with the therapist about the speech and language goals the therapist was working towards with the child. This lack of information meant that the parents had very little idea about which aspects of the speech and language difficulties still needed addressing and what could be done next for their child. Dorothy felt that her son still had a major problem with his speech after a year. But she reported that she had not a chance to discuss with the therapist what would happen then:

She [*the therapist*] hasn't ever said and maybe there isn't another step after this, I don't know, that if he doesn't pick up better . . . we'll do this . . . so maybe there isn't anything else. I don't know. I ain't got a clue.

To add to the uncertainty of a number of the parents, they also felt that they could not approach the therapist on this issue. Dorothy felt awkward about trying to broach the subject with the therapist they had been seeing:

She [*the therapist*] said well, he is improving, improving slowly, very slowly and I sort of felt well I can't sort of question her like, 'If they don't get better any quicker, what then?' 'cos it was sort of questioning her authority like, I'm not qualified, I'm just a mother like, I shouldn't question what she says.

After a year, the parents were looking forward to the future and to continued improvement in their child's speech and language. Some of them accepted that progress might take a while to come about. However, several of the parents highlighted the lack of information about their child's difficulties at that time and what future therapy might entail. Also, the parents' hopes for their child's further progress were sometimes clouded with a number of other worries.

What the parents were worried about

The focus of the parents' concerns at this stage are displayed in Box 7.3.

Box 7.3 Concerns of the parents after 12 months

Their child starting school and coping with the demands made there.

Their child being able to join in with their peer group.

Their child not being different from the other children.

The development of their child's learning and reading skills.

Their being able to receive more therapy if this was necessary.

Starting school

After the 12 month period, many of the children whose parents were interviewed had either started school or were about to start school. Even where
their child's speech and language difficulties were resolving or had resolved,
the parents regarded school as the real testing ground of their child's development. The parents believed that when their children started school, their
speech and language skills had to be good enough for them to be able to learn
effectively, to mix with other children and to be able to make friends with
them. The parents were very aware of the sort of demands that are likely to
be placed on children once they have begun their schooling. They felt
anxious that these huge changes in their child's life might result in further
problems becoming evident:

> I am sort of concerned about him really . . . in the class when you, they ask
> questions . . . he's not going to do it at the moment . . . 'cos he wouldn't know
> what to say . . . so I am a bit concerned about him really. Yeah, how he's going to
> sort of cope really at the school. **Linda**

> It will be interesting to see what happens when he does go to school because we
> may have got it wrong. He may go to school and suddenly totally over-awed with it
> . . . in which case we might start having problems 'cos he might go back to the way
> he was and not communicate. **Ross**

> When you go into proper school . . . and I think that's where his problems are
> going to start when he's trying to be like the other kids and hold conversations and
> they can't understand him and obviously they do take the mickey . . . I think it will

just knock his confidence and he just won't open his mouth even to answer questions in class. **Dorothy**

Joining in with their peer group

Many of the parents expressed concerns that their child's speech and language would get in the way of them mixing with other children at nursery or school and being able to make friends with them:

> He gets so cross and angry especially at playgroup when he plays with his little friends and they don't understand. **Sally**

> He tries to get on well with everybody but I know he doesn't, he tends to stick with, if he got a friend, he'll stick with that particular friend. I don't know, 'cos of his talking maybe he's not mixing so well. **Linda**

> This [*starting nursery*] is now going to be the real test because she's going to have to interact with other children. **Emma**

Not being different from the other children

For many of the parents, starting nursery or school represented a time when any difficulties their child had would become apparent to a wider group of people, outside their circle of family and friends. Therefore, a matter of some concern among the parents was whether or not their child would stand out, among their classmates and teaching staff, as being different because of their speech and language difficulties. The parents were fearful that their child could end up being labelled, rejected and bullied because of their problems:

> I suppose to her she hasn't got a problem but then at that age [*school age*] it can be so easily sort of picked on and like bullied and she don't want anyone to sort of make her feel like she's an alien. I wouldn't like her to think she's different and horrible. **Selina**

> I don't want her to go there [*nursery*] . . . a child that can't speak, 'cos they do get singled out . . . they say adults are evil but children can be just as bad and I don't want her to be treated like she's the one that can't speak and so they don't bother so much with her. **Hayley**

> I was very anxious and still am quite anxious I suppose the way she expresses her frustration at times, will she be labelled as some kind of naughty child . . . and I'm very aware that children can be quite cutting at that age . . . they do make horrible comments about each other. **Isabel**

The development of learning and reading skills

As well as worrying about how their child would get on with others at school, the parents were also anxious that the presence of speech and language difficulties could affect their child's learning and, in particular, how they got on with learning to read:

> I don't really know what will happen with his talking in future but I hope that it will progress and . . . that it will eventually be at a normal level for his age so, without having too much effect on his learning abilities . . . at nursery and school. **Caroline**

> If you can nip it in the bud [*speech and language difficulties*] then all the better for the child. It's got a better prospect 'cos obviously it affects their reading and how they learn as well, so really that speech could hold them back for quite a few years. **Carol**

> I've always had the impression that if you start at the bottom, then you'll always be close to the bottom . . . if we can get him somewhere near the top when he first goes to school then he's more likely to stay there, with more encouragement. **Gary**

Being able to receive more therapy

Many of the children whose parents took part in the interviews were still showing problems after a year. Because of this, their parents felt that more therapy would be needed in the future and were eager to know that this would continue to be provided for their child:

> I'd like it [*the therapy*] to be consistent now, like sort of get into the habit of knowing she's still got to go . . . it's just the back-up to say yes she is doing well. I suppose because we've always had that service there we'll always want to make sure she gets it. **Selina**

This became a source of concern to the parents because they were unsure about how much more help would be offered them and at what point their child might be discharged from speech and language therapy. They felt that they would rely on the therapist to tell them when this time had come, as Emma's statement illustrates:

> I'd like to think that she's up to that scratch but then I don't know who decides that, whether it's the therapist or myself because you could end up as a parent wanting more whereas I think it's better . . . that you've got somebody there

who says, 'No, she's fine', whereas you're like pushing them, pushing them, 'cos you want what's best for them.

Emma felt that she would take the therapist's advice about whether further therapy was necessary or not. However, some parents feared that the therapist might say one thing and they might think another – that the therapist might terminate therapy before they were convinced that the child, or indeed, they were ready for it. At this stage, the parents felt that they were entering unknown territory:

> I wouldn't know now whether he would benefit from any more speech therapy or no . . . I mean I don't make that decision do I really I get advised on that . . . but I mean I don't really know what stage he's at. **Patricia**

In spite of the relationship that may have built up, parents needed a lot of reassurance that their views would be taken into account at all when the decision to end therapy was made. While some parents had felt that they were in partnership with the therapist, they now felt less involved again and that their preferences were not always taken into account:

> He's had a little break [*from therapy*] now, which even that I wasn't that happy about. But she [*the therapist*] said, 'Oh yeah, it'll do him good.' If I'd had my choice I'd have said, 'No I want him to be seen still.' **Amy**

The accounts of the parents paint a vivid picture of their hopes and fears for their children as they approached entry into nursery and school, often with continuing speech and language difficulties. The first part of this chapter has considered in detail the parents' views about their child's progress and outcome after a year. In the last part of the chapter, the research evidence about the course of early speech and language delays and the effects of therapy on the difficulties will be examined.

What is known about the course of early speech and language delays

A number of the parents who took part in the interviews mentioned that other people had told them that their children would eventually grow out of their difficulties and parents might still hear this from family members, friends and professionals. Indeed, a few of the children whose parents were interviewed no longer had any speech and language problems at the end of the year. However, a larger number of children did still have marked difficulties after 12 months. A number of research projects have attempted to follow up children with early speech and language delays to find out what happened to their difficulties over the course of time. The research which has taken place to date confirmed that while some children do grow out of early problems, others do not.

It is suggested that among children with difficulties in learning words and putting words together (expressive language difficulties), as many as 60 per cent may get better without any treatment between the ages of two and three years. However, where children are also experiencing difficulties in understanding language (receptive language difficulties), they run a greater risk of continuing problems. The research project, of which the parent interviews formed a part, found that after a year about three quarters of all the children were still experiencing some level of difficulty in speech and language. This included children with difficulties in understanding and producing language, as well as children with speech sound difficulties. A major problem that speech and language therapists working with young children face is predicting whether and how their difficulties will improve. Very little work has been done in this area. Therefore, therapists still find it very hard to distinguish between the children who are likely to improve and those who are not.

Other research studies have looked at children with early speech and language delays into their school years. There have also been studies which have re-assessed teenage children who had early talking difficulties. So far it has been demonstrated that, whether or not their speech and language have improved, these children may go on to experience difficulties with their performance at school, their behaviour and socialization into their teens. A link between early speech and language delays and later under-achievement in reading and other language-based skills has also been established. As many as 75 per cent of children may go on to have reading problems by the age of eight if they had early language delays.

This suggests that early speech and language delays, even when they get better in the pre-school period, may still leave children at risk of other difficulties once they enter school and beyond. Box 7.4 summarizes the conclusions of the research on the course of speech and language delays to date.

BOX 7.4 RESEARCH CONCLUSIONS ABOUT THE COURSE OF EARLY SPEECH AND LANGUAGE DELAYS

For children with difficulties in learning words and putting words together, up to 60 per cent may get better.

Where children are also having problems with understanding as well as producing language, there is less possibility that they will get better.

Speech and language therapists find it very hard to predict which children are likely to get better and which are not.

A number of projects have shown that children with early delays may go on to experience difficulties with their learning and reading, their behaviour and their social skills.

What is known about the effect of therapy on early speech and language difficulties

A number of the parents whose children received speech and language therapy felt that it had helped to bring about improvements in their children's talking. Other parents were not so sure that the therapy had made any difference. Speech and language therapists, just like these parents, do not know for certain what the course of early talking difficulties is like and also, what the effects of therapy on the difficulties may be. A number of research projects, however, have tried to find out more about what therapy can do for the difficulties. Box 7.5 lists the aspects of the research which will be discussed.

BOX 7.5 ASPECTS OF THE RESEARCH TO BE CONSIDERED

The children who have been involved in the research.

The methods of treatment which have been researched.

Where the research projects have been carried out.

The conclusions of the research to date.

What is not yet known about the effect of therapy.

The children who have been involved in the research

The effects of treatment programmes on children from as young as ten months through to school age have been investigated, although many projects have focused on children in the two to three-and-a-half year age range. The children have come from a range of social backgrounds, where their parents' levels of education and employment have varied enormously. However, a wide range of cultural backgrounds and ethnic groups has not been represented. The types of difficulties experienced by the children which have been investigated to date include difficulties with understanding language (receptive language difficulties), difficulties with learning words and putting words together (expressive language development) and difficulties with producing speech sounds (phonological difficulties).

The methods of treatment which have been researched

A number of different ways of delivering treatment have been researched. These include:

- therapy delivered by a speech and language therapist to children individually
- therapy delivered by the child's parents after training by a speech and language therapist
- therapy delivered by a speech and language therapist to children in groups
- therapy delivered in the form of training sessions for parents to promote their children's speech and language development.

Also, a number of different approaches to intervention have been tested, including:

- the direct teaching of words, sounds and other communication skills to children by encouraging them to copy adult versions
- the indirect teaching of words, sounds and other communication skills, as the opportunity occurs, in a more natural context such as a play setting
- combinations of the above approaches.

Where the research projects have been carried out

Many of the research projects described so far have been carried out in the USA. They have tended to take place in specialist treatment centres where the children have had access to intensive therapy over long periods of time. This means that the projects have often looked at the effects of therapy on the children's difficulties under ideal conditions. For this reason, the therapy the children received in the projects cannot be directly compared with the therapy services offered in community clinics in the UK. This is because in everyday clinic situations therapists may not be able to deliver intensive therapy and they may be using different approaches or combinations of approaches to treatment than the ones which have been investigated. Up until now, only a few studies have attempted to look at speech and language therapy services as they were being delivered in community clinics. Much of the research which has been done, therefore, does not tell us whether the speech and language therapy children usually receive actually 'works'.

The conclusions of the research to date

The research projects which have been carried out so far suggest that:

- Children can benefit from speech and language therapy. The projects have demonstrated improvements in the children's receptive and expressive language and in their use of sounds. Even so, the accounts of some of the parents in this project show that they might still want to delay therapy, even when they think it 'works'.
- When they were receiving therapy for receptive and expressive language difficulties, children benefited as much from the treatment being carried out by their parents, who had received training, as from treatment carried out by the therapist. However, the children with speech sound difficulties did better when therapy was carried out by the therapist. It is uncertain whether it is realistic to ask for the amount of cooperation from other parents which was necessary to bring about these improvements. This is likely to depend upon the other roles, responsibilities and stresses parents are already managing.
- The treatment approaches mentioned above all - direct teaching, indirect teaching and combinations of the two - brought about improvement in the children in the projects.
- There have been no studies, however, which have directly compared therapy given to children at different ages, of different intensity and length, in different locations, using different approaches to treatment.
- The bigger research project, of which these interviews with parents formed a part, concluded that the children who had access to immediate therapy, on average, did not do better than those whose therapy was delayed for a year. The immediate therapy children received, on average, just over five hours of therapy across the year. This is much less therapy than was available to children in many of the other projects and may explain why there were few differences between the immediate and delayed therapy groups. However, this was the amount of therapy that was available to the children at the time of the project in their local clinics. It may be very similar to the therapy provided in other clinics across the UK.
- There is very little information about the longer term effects of therapy and whether or not improvements made in therapy continue afterwards. Projects which have tried to look at this question have been unsuccessful, because many children have dropped out.

A summary of the research findings on the effects of therapy on early speech and language delays is contained in Box 7.6.

> **BOX 7.6 RESEARCH FINDINGS ABOUT THE EFFECTS OF THERAPY ON EARLY SPEECH AND LANGUAGE DELAYS**
>
> The research suggests that speech and language therapy can benefit children with early talking difficulties.
>
> Where benefits have been shown, however, the services received by the children and parents have not always been comparable to those available in community clinics in the UK.
>
> Little is still known about the best ways to tackle early speech and language delays. Speech and language therapists do not know the best timing, the best amount and the best methods of treatment for particular difficulties.
>
> Speech and language therapy may bring about improvements in the difficulties in the short term but the long-term benefit of therapy is uncertain.

What is not yet known about the effect of therapy

A number of questions about speech and language therapy for pre-school children, therefore, still need answering. While it appears that speech and language therapy may 'work' there is not enough information about:

- which children it works for, in terms of the difficulties they have and their backgrounds
- at what age therapy should begin – is it better to treat children when they are very young or to wait until they are older?
- how much therapy is necessary
- for how long it should continue
- what form therapy should take – would individual sessions produce better improvements in children than group sessions? Is it better to teach new words directly or indirectly?

Speech and language therapy needs, therefore, to find better ways of helping children with early speech and language delays. Throughout this book, the parents have spoken of their involvement in their child's speech and language therapy. Therefore, as well as learning how to bring about improvements in the difficulties, finding better ways to help also includes taking into account the opinions of parents about their children's difficulties and the sort of services that fit in with their lives.

This chapter has considered what the parents felt about the course of their children's speech and language delays, the changes that came about and the point they felt their child had reached. It has also presented the research findings which are related to this topic. In the final chapter, the meaning of the parents' accounts will be explored. There will be a re-examination and summing up of some of the themes that have occurred in the book this far. It will also contain a description of the advice that the parents would offer to other parents faced with similar circumstances and suggestions to speech and language therapy departments about changes that could be made in the services they provide to children and their parents.

Summary of the chapter

- A number of the parents who took part in the interviews described the problems and frustrations they came across when coping with their child's speech and language difficulties on an everyday basis.
- All of the parents who were interviewed reported that their child's difficulties had improved in the course of the year.
- The amount of change that had come about varied greatly. Some parents believed their child's difficulties had resolved. Several others believed that the difficulties were on the way to being resolved, while other parents believed that their child was still experiencing significant difficulties.
- When they talked about their child's outcome, some parents said they were happy. A few parents were unhappy about the outcome and one other parent felt very unsure about the outcome.
- The parents spoke about their expectations for the future. Because they had seen improvements come about in the year many of them remained optimistic.
- Several of the parents appreciated how much further their child needed to move on to be able to cope with nursery or school.
- The parents often did not have much idea about what the therapist was aiming to do in their child's speech and language development.
- Even where the children had been receiving regular speech and language therapy the parents reported that they had had little or no discussion with the therapist about any remaining difficulties and how they could be treated after the year.
- After a year the parents were concerned about a number of issues, including their child starting school, their child being able to mix with their peer group and not standing out as being different. They were also concerned about the development of their child's learning and reading skills and provision of future speech and language therapy.
- The research findings relating to the course of early speech and language delays show that many children with difficulties in learning words and putting words together may get better. Where children are also having

problems with understanding as well as producing language, there is less possibility that they will get better. A number of projects have shown that children with early delays may experience difficulties later on.

- Speech and language therapists find it very hard to predict which children are likely to get better and which are not.

- The research findings about the effects of therapy on early speech and language delays suggest that speech and language therapy can benefit children with early talking difficulties. However, where benefits have been shown, services have not always been comparable to those available in community clinics in the UK. Also, speech and language therapy may bring about improvements in the difficulties in the short term but the long-term benefit of therapy is uncertain.

- Little is still known about the best ways to tackle early speech and language delays. Speech and language therapists do not know the best timing, the best amount and the best methods of treatment for particular difficulties.

CHAPTER 8

Understanding the meaning of the parents' accounts

In the previous chapters, the accounts of the parents about their child's difficulties and the speech and language therapy services they received were presented. In telling their stories, a number of themes emerged from the parents again and again. These themes, which spanned all the interviews, when looked at together, provide a summary of the whole experience of the parents from the time when they first became aware that their child was experiencing speech and language difficulties up to the time when they were awaiting their child's entry into school and possible discharge from therapy. They also demonstrate the motivation behind the parents' feelings and actions. These themes will be considered in detail in the first part of the chapter.

At this point, the question may be asked: what is the meaning of these accounts to parents whose children will experience difficulties with talking in the future and to professionals who are concerned with early speech and language delays, like speech and language therapists? Firstly, the possible meaning of these accounts to other parents will be considered. The parents who took part in the interviews revealed varying experiences of and attitudes towards speech and language delays and therapy. Drawing on this range of perspectives and opinions, the advice the parents reported they would give to other parents faced with similar situations to their own will be displayed. Secondly, the meaning of the accounts for professionals working with speech and language-delayed children and their families will be presented. In the last part of the chapter, a discussion of the suggestions made by the parents to improve the way in which speech and language difficulties are dealt with will take place.

The accounts of the parents

To begin, the themes occurring in the parents' accounts which summarized their experience and explained their reasons for thinking and acting as they did are listed in Box 8.1.

BOX 8.1 THEMES SUMMARIZING THE PARENTS' EXPERIENCES DRAWN FROM THEIR ACCOUNTS

The parents' desire for information.

The parents' need for emotional support.

The parents' views about their involvement in the therapy process.

The parents' concerns about their child's future.

'He needs help but why? No one knew, told me why': parents' desire for information

Information about their child's difficulties

The parents' accounts revealed that as soon as they felt something was wrong with their child's speech and language development they began trying to make sense of the difficulties. They speculated about things that might have caused the difficulties in the first place. They wondered if their child's difficulties with talking had arisen because of medical conditions their child had, their own actions in bringing the child up, their family background or because of factors to do with the child him or herself. This often led to the parents feeling puzzled and uncertain because they could not find an explanation. They struggled to understand the difficulties even more when their other children had developed normally and easily. They experienced feelings of guilt because they imagined the problems might be due to things they had done or failed to do.

This early experience of children's difficulties with talking might have been made easier for the parents if they had had appropriate information about early speech and language delays at the time when they were trying to understand their child's problems. But there appeared to be a gap in this instance between the need for information on the part of the parents and what was actually available to them. Many of the parents were eager to find out more about early speech and language delays but did not always know where to look. One parent mentioned looking up information about early speech and language problems in a book dealing with children's development in general. However, no parents mentioned having access to specific leaflets or books about speech and language delay recommended to them by their health visitor, family doctor or speech and language therapist. The parents described their lack of knowledge and information about the difficulties during the time before their child's referral to speech and language therapy. When they had visited the speech and language therapist, some parents did feel that they had been given sufficient explanation about the difficulties and were satisfied with the information they had received.

Even after referral, however, a number of the parents did not always feel informed about the delays and why they came about. At the end of the year when one mother spoke about her son's speech difficulties she still did not feel that she had received an adequate explanation about them.

Information about their child's therapy

Many of the parents reported being given some information about their child's difficulties when they saw the speech and language therapist for the first time and their child was assessed. When their child was allocated to receive immediate therapy, a few parents felt that the information about their child's treatment passed on to them by the therapist had helped them to understand what was taking place in therapy and why. On the other hand, many of the parents reported being told little about what the therapy would entail, how it would be organized and what areas of speech and language would be targeted. One parent opted to pull out of therapy altogether, partly because she did not feel that it was specifically addressing any areas of difficulty with her son. Other parents had expected that particular areas would be worked on in therapy. When they were not, and parents were not given reasons for the targets chosen by the therapist, they continued with therapy reluctantly as they did not feel they were achieving anything by doing so.

Whether or not their children received therapy over the course of the 12 months, a number of the parents were unsure about the point their child had reached at the end of the year. They could not tell themselves whether the progress made by their child meant that his or her speech and language skills were in line with those of other children of a similar age and whether it would be appropriate for therapy to continue. A few parents certainly felt that they did not know what would happen in therapy in the future or even whether future therapy would be offered to them. It is probable that this situation was not helped by the fact that the speech and language therapists themselves may have found it difficult to predict the course of the children's difficulties and whether or not the children would respond to therapy. As the last chapter showed, speech and language therapists continue to be hampered by a lack of research evidence that they can use when making judgements and decisions about children's difficulties.

'At the time we were really concerned for her': parents' need for emotional support

Coping with the difficulties

In the conversations that took place with the parents, they often highlighted the sort of everyday frustrations and upsets they faced when their children had difficulties with talking. Even common occurrences which came about as part of their routine, such as finding out what their child wanted to drink, could end up in a temper tantrum if the child could not make his or her needs known to their parents. In this way, attempts at communication between the parents and their child could become stressful events for parents and children rather than a pleasure. The parents also spoke of the ways in which they had to manage their child's reaction to not being included or understood outside the home and to prepare for the unexpected comments of others. When there is this potential for difficulties in the midst of day-to-day communication, it is easy to understand how their children's talking difficulties caused parents a great deal of anxiety and placed them under considerable pressure.

Feelings of isolation and being 'different'

Before their child was referred to speech and language therapy and up to the time when they were interviewed, parents remarked on how they often felt isolated because of their child's difficulties. Very few of the parents knew other parents whose children had had similar problems and in whom they could confide. This led them to feel as if they were marked out in some way – that they and their child were 'different' from other families. However, many of the parents were relieved that these feelings had lessened over the course of the year and contact with the speech and language therapist had shown them that early talking difficulties were much more common than they had realized. Yet their concerns that their children's difficulties should not leave them feeling isolated and inferior grew once more with the approach of school.

Feelings of uncertainty about attendance at speech and language therapy

Even when it was something that they sought themselves, the referral of their child to speech and language therapy provoked much anxiety in many of the parents. The parents were pleased that if a real problem was identified by the speech and language therapist something could be done about it. They hoped that their child's problems would turn out to be mild. However, they were also concerned that their initial attendance at speech and language therapy might confirm their worst fears about the difficulties.

Added to this, the parents often did not know what to expect of speech and language therapy and the therapist. They were anxious that the situation would be too much for their child to cope with and that the demands placed on their child in the assessment might be too great. Many of the parents were relieved to find that attendance at speech and language therapy was relaxed and reassuring and their feelings of anxiety soon disappeared. For a couple of

parents, however, the anxiety they had felt leading up to their first attendance continued beyond this point. One mother could not see what the aim
of her son's therapy was and she explained how this prompted her to worry
more. She described how a lack of information from the therapist left her
wondering whether he had more of a problem than she had been told about.

'It still comes down to what happens at home': parents' views about their involvement in the therapy process

Helping parents to help children

Many of the parents appreciated early on that they would need to take a role in
the therapy their child received. They understood that however much time
they were able to spend with the therapist, work with the children on areas
pointed out by the therapist would still need to take place at home. Even when
some of the parents had not anticipated taking a part in the therapy, they were
happy to involve themselves in the process, to receive help from the therapist
so that they could help their child themselves. For some of the parents, this
arrangement worked well and they felt happy about the speech and language
therapy homework they were doing. However, a number of the parents
indicated that while they had tried to get involved with the process of therapy,
they found it very difficult to do so. To be able to deliver therapy to their
children, they felt in need of guidance and support from the therapist. Several
parents mentioned that they had not received enough ideas and information to
carry out treatment at home. Other parents complained of insufficient undis-
turbed time with the therapist when they could go over the advice and
activities recommended by the therapist to help their child. For a number of
years, speech and language therapy has spoken about the 'empowerment' of
parents – equipping parents to deliver therapy to their children. However, to
these parents empowerment was only possible when knowledge and back-up
from the speech and language therapist was easily available to them.

Wanting to do the right thing

The accounts of the parents show that they were keen to do the 'right thing'
for their child. This meant that as soon as they became aware that their child
might have a difficulty with talking they involved their health visitor and
sought advice about what they could do. When their health visitor recommended referral to speech and language therapy, all but one of the parents
interviewed agreed for this to go ahead. Two other parents acted in different
ways when they suspected difficulties – one mother referred her son herself
and the other went along to her GP for the referral to be made. When the

parents attended speech and language therapy for the first time they were asked whether they would be willing to participate in a research project, all agreed. Later on when they were interviewed the parents described how, by taking part in the research, they would be giving something back to society and contributing to the development of knowledge which could help children in the future.

The parents demonstrated their positive response to their child's difficulties and accepted whatever help they were offered in dealing with the problems. At the same time, however, several of the parents felt that the speech and language therapy service they had received had been less than positive towards them. These parents were disappointed because they felt that their perspectives, circumstances and needs were not always taken into account by the speech and language therapist they saw. When difficulties arose, the parents often did not feel that they could question the therapist and attempt to resolve them. This sometimes led the parents to become disillusioned with the therapy and to one parent withdrawing from it altogether. In the interviews, these parents tried to avoid sounding negative about the speech and language therapy service, even though they were not satisfied with what they had received. One mother explained that she did not want to sound ungrateful, although she felt that therapy had not made any difference to her child's difficulties.

'I don't know if he's going to improve in weeks, months or whether it's going to take a long time': parents' concerns for their child's future

Even before referral to speech and language therapy, the parents described how anxious they were that, in spite of their children's difficulties, they would be able to join in with what was going on around them, mix with other children and take advantage of the play and learning experiences that came their way. The almost constant comparing of their child, in spite of their guilt about doing so, to their brothers, sisters and peer group increased the worry and pressure felt by parents. Over the course of the year, as the children made progress, parents' worries came and went. However, by the end of the year, the parents were starting to highlight afresh all the concerns they felt over their children starting school, being able to mix with their peer groups and not standing out from the rest of the children. They were also worried about their children's learning in the future and how the talking difficulties might affect this and whether or not they would still be able to receive therapy in the future.

The conversations with parents underlined the fact that their hopes and fears for their children had not ended, but were set to continue for a long time. Normality was certainly a goal for some of the children, although their parents remarked how uncertain they were about what 'normal' children's speech and language were like at the age their child was. A few parents had started the slow and painful acceptance that normality would be very hard, if not impossible, to achieve. Thus the worry and uncertainty experienced by parents when they first became aware of their child's difficulties were not always quickly replaced with feelings of hope and confidence that the problems would resolve. At this time, as at the beginning of their contact with speech and language therapy, parents were eager to take up the help that was on offer to them and wanted to ensure that the therapy they felt had benefited their child would continue.

The meaning of parents' accounts to other parents

The parents who took part in the interviews came from a range of backgrounds and held a range of views about speech and language delays and therapy. At the end of the year, they had gained information and under-standing about their child's early speech and language delays and what speech and language therapy could offer them. For these reasons, they were asked what they might tell other parents faced with similar problems in their own children. The types of advice the parents said they would pass on are listed in Box 8.2.

BOX 8.2 ADVICE THE PARENTS WOULD PASS ON TO OTHER PARENTS

Making practical suggestions for helping children.

Highlighting the need to involve professionals where problems were suspected.

Raising awareness of speech and language delays and therapy.

Practical suggestions

After their own experiences, the parents understood how eagerly other parents might wish for practical advice and suggestions to help cope with the speech and language difficulties. For that reason, a number of parents said that they would pass on leaflets they had been given during the project listing concrete ideas for helping speech and language development:

> I mean if I had the leaflets and that here I'd sort of sit down with them and show them that and I'd probably tell them things like I do with her. **Monica**

Others mentioned that they would demonstrate to parents the ways in which they were helping their own child and give ideas for games and activities:

> I'd sort of show them some of the games you were taught, I was taught to do with him, things like that. **Amy**

Several others said they would be keen to show other parents how they could encourage their child to make choices in everyday communication situations and how the parents should use techniques like repeating back to their child words they had said incorrectly:

> Just give him a choice of words . . . would you rather have juice or Coke? **Linda**

> Be patient with them and repeat everything back to them clearly and the right way. **Carol**

One parent was even more specific. She strongly recommended building up a scrapbook of pictures tailored to the child's life that could then be used for communication purposes:

> I'd also tell them [*other parents*] do the book like I done . . . do the faces that they see every day . . . take pictures of people, cut them up, stick them in a book. **Hayley**

Recalling their own struggles, they urged other parents to show patience and a positive attitude towards their child:

> Concentrate on the positive things that they can do and not criticize too much the stuff that they can't do. **Caroline**

While they understood all too well the feelings of frustration, they wanted other parents to encourage their child as much as they could and to persevere with their child's attempts at communications. The parents described how comparing their child with others had led them into a vicious circle where comparison had led to worry and worry had made them compare even more. They admitted that it was very tempting to make comparisons with other children but believed that this was a negative practice which made things worse not better:

> I suppose you always feel you gotta keep up with other people, there's no need really. The only thing is, don't worry about other people, it's easy to say but it's hard to do. **Selina**

While they were happy in the interviews to recount possible advice they would give, many of the parents remained shy about the possibility of advising others. Several of the parents felt that the issue of advising others was a matter of some debate, as other parents might class it as interference and each person's experience was likely to be different. They also wished to avoid being possibly labelled as a 'know-all' by other parents:

> I would probably tell them of my experience and how, this is contentious, isn't it? It's difficult because this is where the controversy starts 'cos one parents says how they've got on with their child, then somebody else says, and you say which way . . . this is why I wouldn't say it to other people unless they actually asked. **Emma**

> I'd hate to give advice 'cos it sounds as if you know it all, doesn't it? **Andrea**

In spite of their uncertainty, the practical suggestions that came from parents stressed their understanding of the need for support, both practical and moral, when confronting children's developmental difficulties. They also demonstrated that the provision of advice from one parent to another might be an effective way of helping families.

Highlighting the need to involve professionals

All of the parents who were interviewed strongly advised other parents to involve and seek help from professionals like health visitors and speech and language therapists if they had a suspicion that their child's talking was not developing as it should. The older the child was, the more urgent the parents considered referral to speech and language therapy to be:

> I did have a friend and I told her to refer herself to a speech therapist . . . I mean I suppose it depends on the age of the child in fairness. **Sally**

> I mean I have got friends who feel very anxious when their child isn't talking at the age of 18 months . . . I would probably offer reassuring words at that age. I suppose if their speech had been as limited as hers at maybe round the two mark then . . . I would probably also suggest that they go and talk to their health visitor. **Isabel**

Surprisingly, even the parents who had been unenthusiastic about therapy still recommended following this course of action:

> I wouldn't advise anybody not to go for speech therapy because I don't think it does any harm and I think it could maybe do some good, for some children, depending on what type of speech therapy they get. **Caroline**

> I wouldn't turn around and say to anyone, 'Oh it's a waste of time', because in some cases it isn't, you know. I'm not knocking speech therapy altogether because I wouldn't do that, 'cos there are kids quite obviously that will benefit from it. **Dorothy**

Many of the parents felt that their emphasis at this stage would be to reassure parents but at the same time they would try to persuade them to get any possible problems investigated, including their child's hearing. Several of the parents judged that their children's hearing problems had been connected to their speech and language difficulties and felt, therefore, that it was extremely important to establish whether hearing loss might be contributing to the difficulties. The overwhelming message from the parents was try not to worry, do not try to cope alone and involve professionals to check the problems:

> I would probably say it's all going to be fine in time . . . and at the same time I do think that you need sort of therapist and the medical sort of support to keep an eye on these things. **Wendy**

Raising awareness of speech and language delays

The parents could recall their own hazy ideas about speech and language delays and what might cause them. For that reason, they felt that they would seek to raise awareness among other parents by speaking of their own experiences:

> I mean you must find out what the problem is . . . and I would tell them what we've been through and encourage them to do all they can to help. **Fiona**

The parents were aware also that some parents might be reluctant for their children to be referred to speech and language therapy. Remembering their own preconceptions and expectations, they acknowledged that parents might be worried about attendance at speech and language therapy. However, they felt that they could use their own story in a positive way to highlight that there should be no shame attached to attending speech and language therapy and that seeking qualified help was the right step to take:

> I certainly wouldn't mind telling anybody how we've gotten on with it and even try to convince them I suppose that it is really is not anything to, don't know if shame's the right word, but some people do feel ashamed by these things . . . that because they've got this not quite perfect child. **Patricia**

The meaning of parents' accounts to speech and language therapists

In the interviews, parents were asked what changes they could suggest which would make life with a child with early speech and language delays easier. The experiences the parents had had crystallized into specific suggestions for changes which have implications for professionals who work with speech and language-delayed children and their families. Their suggestions are displayed in Box 8.3.

BOX 8.3 SUGGESTIONS FOR IMPROVEMENTS IN SPEECH AND LANGUAGE THERAPY MADE BY THE PARENTS

The frequency of therapy.

The format of therapy.

The relationship between the families and the speech and language therapist.

Help offered by the speech and language therapist specifically for parents.

The frequency of therapy

One of the most frequent suggestions from the parents about what would help children with speech and language difficulties was to increase the frequency of therapy:

> I'd say the only thing that I'd moan about is that I wish the sessions were more often. **Amy**

> If it could be more frequent then I think that would improve things. **Gary**

The parents whose children's therapy was delayed also wanted more frequent contact with the speech and language therapist. Carol had been happy to monitor her little boy's speech and language and not go ahead immediately with therapy. However, she still felt that a six month gap between re-assessments was too long:

> I would have preferred a less waiting time and I would have been slightly concerned . . . if we would have had to have waited longer.

On the other hand, Sandra reported that she would have preferred more clearly defined bursts of therapy taking place over a short period of time. Instead she felt that her son's therapy dragged on and on:

> I don't know where she [*the therapist*] was heading to. She should have said therefore to me that we are doing three sessions of this and then we will progress to this and that, because it just seemed so endless and I couldn't see the progression.

While many of the parents would have appreciated more frequent sessions, they felt that short sessions, especially when their child was being assessed, would be better:

> I mean the sessions were . . . maybe a bit lengthy. There was a lot to fit in but they could be shortened slightly. **Wendy**

The format of therapy

The parents had often developed their own ways of coping with their children's difficulties over the course of the year. But, as Caroline's statement shows, they were also keen to share their experience with other parents and to learn from them:

> I don't know whether it might be an idea to maybe do it in groups or something. Have a group of children and a group of parents, therefore the parents could speak to each other and get advice or ideas from each other.

Several parents also questioned whether providing therapy for the children in groups might be a good way to help them:

> Have a group of children . . . then maybe it would be more structured 'cos they'd be doing a group activity type thing that was very specific towards learning words and language. **Caroline**

> I suppose also I do wonder . . . about maybe some sort of form of group work with the child . . . a child who's at her age now, who's coming up to four, you know, can often be influenced by peers and would enjoy that kind of session. **Isabel**

A number of the parents spoke of how difficult they found it to take down ideas and advice during therapy sessions when their child was present. They then found it difficult to carry out therapy at home because they could not always remember the suggestions that had been made to them. For this reason, a few parents suggested that parents could be seen by the speech and language therapist without their children being present, either individually or in groups:

> I think if you're going to talk to the parent about things, I think you might as well tell the parent that the children are just there for a play for a start and just or, not to bring them, if the parent doesn't want to and to talk with the parents directly and try and reinforce things at home. **Sandra**

> It would almost be a good idea to have the mums and the therapists together at a separate occasion . . . to go through the problems discussing how . . . to help the children with the problems. I don't know . . . how easy that would be. **Fiona**

One parent also queried whether it would be better for children to be seen without their parents in the room. Dorothy felt that her son would find it easier to respond to therapy and would concentrate better if she were not around for all of the session:

> Once the child has got to know the speech therapist I think they should be seen on their own. **Dorothy**

Several parents wondered whether more therapy for children should be provided in the child's home. They felt that children were less relaxed in clinic than in their own environment and therefore less likely to take things in:

> I don't know maybe doing it in the home more often might help because I know when he went there [*the clinic*] he was totally different . . . he goes shy or he goes a bit quiet . . . whereas at home he's more himself because he's in surroundings that he knows. **Kate**

> I do wonder sometimes about doing work with children within the home environment . . . whether that would be more conducive to holding a child's attention, especially if they're a bit younger where they're around familiar things, familiar toys. **Isabel**

The relationship between the families and the speech and language therapist

A number of the parents commented on how the relationship between themselves and the speech and language therapist could have been improved. Caroline felt that the therapy her son received was not made personal to him and his family and that it was not reflective of his home life. She felt the therapist focused on his performance on test results and whether his development was in line with children of his own age:

> I think it [*the therapy*] was just concentrating on what children of that age should be able to do rather than . . . but those things didn't seem to be necessarily linked with home and school and life.

Another parent had felt patronized by the speech and language therapist she saw. She explained that she had experienced reading and writing difficulties at school herself and sometimes could not follow written instructions. Also, as a single parent, she was not able to afford games recommended by the therapist. For these reasons, she did not think that the therapist had taken her circumstances into account when working with her and her child. She considered that this was essential if parents and therapists were going to work well together:

> I think they should understand you and your child before they turn round and say, 'You should be doing this', 'You should be doing that', 'cos you may not be able to do it. **Hayley**

Another of the parents felt that the speech and language therapist had to be honest with parents and tell them exactly how their children were getting on:

> . . . being honest with the parents. Like I said she [*the therapist*] assessed him but it wasn't her that told me he was a year behind in his development with his speech. **Dorothy**

Help offered by the speech and language therapist specifically for parents

The parents also made suggestions about what help they would have welcomed for themselves. Several of the parents called for more written information and applicable ideas so that they could help their children more effectively:

> I think . . . a bit more of a practical . . . written piece of information . . . the only information that we had at the beginning . . . just didn't seem applicable enough. **Fiona**

> I've always believed that more information is better and if you can get more information frequently, yeah. **Gary**

At the time when they first saw the speech and language therapist, one father remarked that he would have found information on possible causes of speech and language delays helpful:

> It would have been nice if just to have had some sort of explanation of the possi-bilities . . . perhaps the causes of speech impediments, so that we could think well it's not that, it's not that, could be that and could bear that in mind. **Ross**

Besides more written information, the parents commented how they were also in need of more reassurance than they actually received. Speech and language delays in their children often provoked worry, insecurity and fear in the parents. Emotional support from the speech and language therapist, therefore, was very important to them in helping them cope with the difficulties:

> I had realized that he was a bit slow but I think a little pat on the back saying, 'Well don't worry, it does take time, not all of them do things the same way at the same time' . . . something like that might have been more appropriate. **Sandra**

In addition to providing reassurance, Sandra also pointed out the need for therapists to provide parents with clear explanations of what is worked on and why. Because this information was not shared with her, Sandra became even more concerned about what could be wrong with her son when the therapist did not attempt to tell her what was happening in therapy:

> I was never really quite sure when she was meant to be helping me or when she was meant to be helping him . . . I had to dig around a bit to find out what she was even meaning by it . . . I think it should be very upfront and very explained and more set out.

What could be done to help children with early speech and language delays

In the interviews the parents spoke of the ways in which they struggled to come to terms with their child's early difficulties. They sometimes talked about their struggle to receive the help they felt their child needed. Having had this experience, they felt able to make suggestions about changes in the way speech and language therapy could work with them and their children. But the parents also drew attention to the struggles they faced outside their own family and the speech and language therapy service. They highlighted the need for more profound changes in the way early speech and language delays are viewed by society as a whole.

When speech and language difficulties arose in their children, the parents showed how they wanted to do all they could to help and wanted the involvement and support of professionals. Selina spoke of the stigmatizing attitudes of others towards children like her daughter who experienced early difficulties with talking. But she also pointed out that the needs of children like hers might not seem as important as those of children with more obvious problems:

> A lot of people, I think, just presume because you're not disabled you don't need, deserve it.

As far as Selina was concerned, there was nothing wrong with the speech and language therapy services she and her child received. In her mind, the problems lay in the attitudes of others towards children's speech and language difficulties. To help them and their families, she felt that there needed to be an increase in the public awareness and understanding of the difficulties they face:

> You've got to . . . explain yourself all the time to some people and you think, 'Oh I shouldn't have to do this.' If they were more aware of what the services are for then they would sort of know . . . it's people's awareness of things, I think is the problem, not the actual service, it's other people.

Summary of the chapter

- A number of themes recurred when the parents recounted their experiences of their children's early speech and language delays and the speech and language therapy they received.
- At all stages of the process, the parents talked about their desire for information about the delays themselves and the treatment they received.
- The parents also spoke of their need for emotional support as they attempted to cope with their child's difficulties.
- The parents' views of their involvement in the therapy process did not always coincide with those of the therapist. While the parents wanted to help their children they needed greater guidance and support from the therapist to do this.
- The parents' concerns about their child's future were very apparent in the interviews and some of the parents were aware that their child's problems might continue.
- The parents talked about the advice they might pass on to other parents faced with similar problems. This included practical suggestions for helping their children, highlighting the need to involve professionals

where problems were suspected and to raise awareness of speech and language delays and therapy.

- The parents also made a number of suggestions about ways in which speech and language therapy services for children could be improved.
- Increasing the frequency of therapy and changing the format of therapy were the most common suggestions.
- Some parents hoped for better relationships between families and the speech and language therapist, where the therapist could be more responsive to the child and their families as individuals.
- The parents suggested specific ways in which they would have liked help from the speech and language therapist.
- Outside the speech and language therapy service, the attitudes of others to children's speech and language difficulties and therapy were criticized. It was felt that there should be greater public awareness and understanding of the difficulties.

Appendix

Background to the project

The Speech and Language Therapy Effectiveness with Pre-school children (STEP) project, of which the parent interview study formed a part, ran from August 1995 to July 1999. It was funded by the Research and Development Directorate of the NHS Executive South West, and carried out by the Speech and Language Therapy Research Unit, Frenchay Hospital, Bristol. The research team was made up of three research speech and language therapists and a medical statistician, who designed, conducted and disseminated the project. The wider project aimed to explore the impact of the community-based speech and language therapy provision available at the time for pre-school children in two health care trusts in the Bristol area. The parents' views of their children's difficulties and the speech and language therapy service they received were also investigated as part of the project.

The idea for the parent interview study arose from two main sources. Firstly, in the last two decades there has been a particular increase in the involvement of parents in monitoring their children's health and development. Also, parents have been expected to participate more and more in early intervention programmes when their children have experienced developmental difficulties. This corresponds to an increasing emphasis, in the wider context of the National Health Service, on shared clinical decision-making, where clients and professionals discuss and negotiate what form treatment should take. Little research has been conducted, however, into looking at parents' views of this involvement in their children's health care.

Secondly, within the National Health Service, there is growing recognition of the importance of patients' perceptions and opinions about treatments received. Gauging the 'acceptability' of a treatment to clients is becoming an essential component in measuring the outcomes of treatments and investigating their effectiveness. Successive governments have recommended the involvement of clients in assessing the quality of health care. For that reason, the importance of taking client views into account in the evaluation of health services is being stressed in research into health care services. Few projects have been designed to investigate this.

Because of these influences the interview component of the project was designed with two main aims in mind. First, it aimed to explore the parents' views and opinions about their children's speech and language delays and their involvement in the monitoring and treatment of these difficulties. Second, the project aimed to explore the acceptability of the speech and language therapy services received by the parents and their children.

The methodology used in the project

Because of the aims of the project, a qualitative methodology was the one that was considered to be the most appropriate when exploring the views of parents about the speech and language difficulties experienced by their children and the therapy services available to them. In-depth interviewing provides one method of exploring the experiences, beliefs and opinions of people who form the subject of the research. Very importantly, it provides an opportunity for the respondent to raise their own issues and concerns, as well as respond to those brought up by the researcher. This form of interviewing also allows detailed exploration of these issues and the interviewer can take on expressions and forms of language used by the respondents themselves. While remaining flexible, the method is still systematic and rigorous. The planning of the project ensured that the choice of respondents, the conduct of the interviews and the analysis of the resulting material could stand up to close methodological scrutiny.

The respondents

While a commitment is being shown in health services research to giving a voice to all users of services, it was not possible to investigate the perspective of the children themselves. The oldest of them was still only four-and-a-half years old at the time the interviews were carried out. However, the interest of parents in their children's development and their increasing role in therapy made it crucial to gain an understanding of their perspective. At the beginning of the interviewing process, it was intended that roughly equal groups of parents of children allocated to immediate therapy and delayed therapy should be selected. During the course of the interviews, this proposed sample underwent some change, as is often the case in this type of exploratory work. The decision was made to follow up as many as possible of the parents who opted to switch their children from the delayed therapy group to the immediate treatment group. Every attempt was made to interview as many of these parents as possible within the time-frame allowed for data collection, but two were not followed up. In one case, the child had been diagnosed as autistic and for that reason was quite different from the rest of the children involved in the project. In the other case, the mother was experiencing health problems, which made it difficult for her to be interviewed. In a similar way, every attempt was made to identify and interview the other parents whose children had been allocated to the immediate treatment group and then failed to attend appointments and/or comply with treatment. The sample was also designed to include parents from different backgrounds, parents of children of differing ages, with differing extent of difficulties.

At their child's 12 month re-assessment all parents whose children took part in the project were asked by the research speech and language therapist assessing their child if they would consent to be interviewed. During this session they were given an information leaflet to explain the interview process. If they were subsequently chosen to be interviewed, they were contacted by letter, within a month of their child leaving the project. They were then contacted by telephone several days later to arrange a time for the interview, if they still consented. Only one parent contacted at this stage did not wish to be interviewed. All the interviews were carried out in the respondents' homes.

Altogether, the parents of 20 children participated in the project. Of this number, 17 were conducted with the mother alone. In the other three interviews, the mother was joined by her husband, in each case the child's father. Two of these fathers, due to the nature of their work commitments, had taken an active role in their child's involvement in speech and language therapy and for this reason wanted to be present at the interview and to contribute their views and opinions. Every attempt was made in the course of these interviews to check where the opinions of these parents might differ from each other. During the analysis, any discrepancies between the views of mother and father were highlighted.

The parents were purposively selected to make sure that a range of circumstances and backgrounds was represented. These were as follows:

Allocation

The sample comprised the parents of six children allocated to immediate therapy, six children allocated to delayed therapy and eight children originally allocated to delayed therapy but who started receiving treatment before the 12 month period.

Gender

The parents of 15 boys and five girls took part in the interviews.

Age

The sample was selected to ensure that the experiences of parents with younger and older children were represented. The youngest child whose parent was interviewed was three years, three months and the oldest child was four years, six months. The age distribution of the children was as follows:

Number of children in each age band
Up to three years, six months   4
Between three years, seven months and four years   8
Between four years, one month and four years, six months   8

Severity of the child's difficulties after 12 months

A range of severity of difficulties was achieved, including the parents of children whose difficulties had resolved and those whose problems were severe and persisting.

Number of children in each severity band
Problems resolved or resolving   5
Delayed in speech only   6
Delayed in speech and language   9

Employment

The parents interviewed also covered a broad range of employment categories. Approximately one fifth of the sample of parents were not in employment, a fifth were doing unskilled or manual jobs, a further two fifths were doing work of a skilled or technical nature, while another fifth were in professional employment.

Ethnicity

Children learning two or more languages at home were not included in the original project. Thus it was not possible to sample the experiences of people from different ethnic groups.

Location

All the respondents were living in the Greater Bristol area at the time they were interviewed. Some parents were from urban locations, others from rural ones.

The topic guide

A topic guide was used in each of the interviews to ensure that all the issues were systematically covered. The author of this book, who carried out all the interviews with the parents, followed the topic guide but was flexible in listening to and following up new issues and concerns voiced by the parents. The topic guide was designed to include a number of different issues:

- What led up to referral of their child to speech and language therapy and their feelings about this
- The child's first appointment and the assessment process
- The parents' previous experiences and preconceptions about speech and language therapy
- The child's talking at that time, the parents' feelings about it and how they were coping with the difficulties at the time
- The parents' ideas regarding the cause of early speech and language delays
- The parents' feelings about the group to which their child was allocated
- The parents' views of the effects of the group
- The roles and responsibilities of parents and speech and language therapy
- The parents' views of their child's talking after 12 months
- The parents' feelings about the re-assessments which happened as part of the project and their involvement in a research project
- The parents' views about the future – what would happen to their children
- Advice the parents would give to other parents in the same situation
- How the parents felt living with early speech and language delays could be made easier.

Before the interviews took place, the author received training in in-depth interviewing. Two pilot interviews with other parents whose children were taking part in the research were carried out.

Analysis of the interview material

Each of the interviews was tape-recorded, with the permission of the respondent and then transcribed word for word. At all stages of the process, the details of the respondents were treated in the strictest confidence by the author. In this book and in other publications, names and some personal circumstances have been altered to maintain the anonymity of the respondents. The interviews were analysed in five sets of four. Thus, analysis of four interviews took place, before the next set of four interviews began. The data were analysed according to the 'Framework' method, developed by the National Centre for Social Research (Ritchie and Spencer 1994). In this project, the initial stage of the analysis involved the drawing up of a system of codes to describe all the themes and issues that occurred in the initial set of interviews. The interview transcripts were then classified and coded. The next stage of the analysis consisted of the division of the text according to theme and the transfer of these pieces of text onto individual theme charts interview by interview. In this way, it was possible to view respondents' opinions across a number of sequential themes and also to compare the views of respondents within a certain theme.

Reference

Ritchie J, Spencer L (1994) 'Qualitative data analysis for applied policy research.' In Bryman A, Burgess R (eds) Analysing Qualitative Data. London: Routledge.

More about the parents who took part in the interviews

In order to protect the identity of the interview respondents, the names by which they are referred to in the book have been anonymized and some of their personal details have been changed.

Sally

Sally's son had been allocated to the delayed therapy group. At the end of their involvement in the project, the child was four years old and was still experiencing significant speech problems, which continued to affect his intelligibility. The child's family was very aware of the difficulties being experienced by the child and felt that there had not been much improvement during the 12 months. The mother felt that early therapy would have been helpful. The family was made up of the mother, father, elder brother and child. The elder brother had experienced no speech or language difficulties at all. The child's mother had had some prior knowledge of speech and language therapy as she worked as a school nurse. The child's father was employed as a landscape gardener.

Amy

Amy's son had been allocated to the immediate therapy group. At the end of their involvement in the project, the child was four years, four months. He was still experiencing some speech problems. The child's family accepted that he needed to improve but the mother felt that therapy had helped a lot. The family was made up of the mother, father, child and younger sister. The younger sister was not experiencing any speech or language difficulties at all. Her mother felt that she was learning to talk very quickly when compared with her son's progress. Both parents worked – the mother was a health care assistant in a local hospital and the father was a decorator. There had been some prior experience of speech and language therapy within the wider family.

Caroline

Caroline's son had been allocated to the immediate therapy group. At the end of their involvement in the project, he was three years, three months and was still experiencing both speech and language difficulties. Caroline felt that her child had significant difficulties and that the progress the child had made over the 12 months had not been due to therapy at all. This parent's attitude towards therapy was that she 'couldn't see the point' of it. The family was made up of the mother and two children, with a friend of the mother living with the family. The child's elder sister had not had any speech or language difficulties. The mother worked as a swimming instructor. She had no prior experience of speech and language therapy.

Linda

Linda's son had been allocated to the delayed therapy group originally. He had switched to the immediate therapy group, at the request of his mother at the six month point. At the end of their involvement in the project, the child was three years, seven months and was still experiencing speech and language difficulties, which were recognized by the family. The mother felt that progress achieved would have not been as much without therapy. The family comprised the mother, father and two children. The child's elder sister had had no problems with talking. Both parents worked – Linda was employed as an office clerk while her husband was a park attendant. There was no prior experience of speech and language therapy.

Bernadette and Ross

This was the first opportunity to interview a father along with a mother. The mother, in this case, had wanted her husband to be present for the interview because he had been involved in taking their child to assessment sessions as well. Their son had been allocated to the delayed therapy group and at the end of their involvement in the project was four years, six months. He had no remaining speech or language difficulties. Both parents were pleased with the progress the child had made without therapy and said that they had never been particularly worried. The family was made up of the mother, father, an older brother and sister and the child. The child's sister had experienced speech difficulties and the mother had taken this child to speech and language therapy. Both parents were working – the mother was employed as a shop assistant while the father was a social worker.

Emma

Emma's daughter had been allocated to the delayed therapy group. At the end of their involvement in the project, the child was three years, three months and still had some speech and language difficulties, which were recognized by the family. The mother felt that waiting had given the child chance to develop without therapy and that progress had been made. She also believed that her child could not have coped with earlier intervention. She was very happy at that point that intensive therapy was underway. The family was made up of the mother, father and two children. The child's younger brother was on the point of being referred to speech and language therapy for language delay, which was not a worry for the mother. Both parents worked. Emma was a nursery nurse while her husband was a fire officer. They had had some previous experience of speech and language therapy, as the father had attended as a child. He was able to recall very little about this experience.

Sandra

Sandra's son had been allocated to the immediate therapy group. At the end of their involvement in the project, the child was four years old. At the time when the interview with his mother took place, he had actually started school. The child was still experiencing some speech difficulties, although the child's mother did not see this as a problem. This mother had not wanted the child to be referred to speech and language therapy and had been disappointed when she had been allocated to receive treatment. She had attended therapy for a while but decided to drop out because it was a 'waste of time'. The family was made up of the mother, father, one older sister, the child and one younger brother. The older sister had experienced no talking difficulties early on and the younger brother was developing without any difficulties. The mother did not work outside the home. The father worked as a computer programmer. There had been no prior experiences of speech and language therapy.

Selina

Selina's daughter had been allocated to the immediate therapy group. At the end of their involvement in the project, the child was three years, three months and was still experiencing delay in speech and language, which the family recognized. The mother felt that the child wouldn't have improved as much without therapy. The family was made up of the mother, father, the child and one younger sister, whose speech and language development had so far given no cause for concern. Both parents were out of work and both had had personal experience of speech and language therapy when younger. Selina pointed out that the therapy received by her daughter had been different from that she had received. (Her own therapy had taken place when she was at school and had focused on speech sound work.)

Carol

Carol's son had been allocated to the delayed therapy group and at the end of their involvement in the project was three years, nine months old. He was still experiencing significant speech problems, which the family acknowledged. The mother was happy that intensive therapy was now going ahead although she felt that the child had made progress without it. She felt that earlier on the child may not have been able to cope with the demands of therapy. The family was made up of the mother, father and two children. The child's elder sister had had no difficulties in learning to talk. The mother worked on a part-time basis as a shop assistant, while the father's employment was as a bricklayer. There had been no prior experience of speech and language therapy.

Fiona

Fiona's son had been allocated in the beginning to the delayed therapy group but the mother, after a few weeks of waiting only, had wanted to change group. At the end of their involvement in the project, the child was aged four years, one month. The child's difficulties had almost resolved, with the exception of some discrete language and social-interactive difficulties, which his parents were aware of. The mother felt that the child would not have made as much progress without therapy and would not have been prepared to wait for therapy any longer than she did. The family was made up of the mother, father, child and a younger brother, who was still a very young baby at the time of the interview. The mother was not working outside the home and the father was employed as an accountant. There had been no prior experience of speech and language therapy.

Patricia

Patricia's son had been allocated to the immediate therapy group. At the end of their involvement in the project, the child was four years, three months and had been at school for about two and a half months. The child's speech and language difficulties were on the way to resolving, although the parents were not concerned about the progress he still needed to make. The mother was positive about the therapy that her child had received and had also attended therapy for her two older sons, whose speech and language development had eventually come about successfully. The family comprised the mother, father, the two older brothers and the child. The mother worked part-time as a dressmaker while the father worked as a salesman.

Hayley

Hayley's daughter had originally been allocated to the delayed therapy group but the mother had wanted to change group at the six month point, possibly after the nursery her daughter was attending had applied some pressure for her to do so. The child was aged three years, three months at the end of their involvement in the project. She continued to experience serious delays in her speech and language. Hayley said that if her child had been making some progress she would have been happy to continue to wait. At the 12 month point, she was not sure how much therapy had actually helped but was set to continue her attendance with the child. The family consisted solely of the mother and the child - there were no brother and sisters. The mother was not working at the time of the interview. There had been some prior experience of speech and language therapy in the wider family.

Andrea

Andrea's son had been allocated to the delayed therapy group. At the end of their involvement in the project, the child was three years, eleven months. His early speech and language difficulties had resolved and the family was delighted by the child's progress. Andrea said that she had never been hugely concerned and that she had been happy to wait and be monitored. The family consisted of the mother, father and child - there were no brothers or sisters. Both parents worked as office clerks. There had been no prior experience of speech and language therapy.

Jacky and Gary

This was the second interview which gave the opportunity to interview a father and a mother. The child had originally been allocated to the delayed therapy group but had changed group at the request of the parents before the six month point. At the end of their involvement in the project, the child was aged four years, five months and his speech and language difficulties appeared to be resolving. His parents felt that he was making progress, but they were very pleased that they had opted to change and put a lot of the child's progress down to therapy. The family was made up of the mother, father, child and one younger brother, who was not experiencing any talking difficulties. The mother did not work outside the home and the father managed a transport company. They had no prior knowledge of speech and language therapy.

Marianne

Marianne's son had had originally been allocated to the delayed therapy group but Marianne had wanted to change group after a wait of six months. At the end of their involvement in the project, the child was three years, eleven months and was considered by nursery staff and the speech and language therapist he was seeing to have a specific language impairment. For that reason, it was thought likely that he would need to attend a special language unit. The mother seemed to appreciate that the child still had a lot of problems but did not appear to be aware of the long-term nature of her son's difficulties. She felt that therapy had helped the child and was glad that she had decided to swap. The family was made up of the mother, child and one younger brother, who was learning to talk normally. At the time of the interview, the mother's partner was living with the family. The mother did not work outside the home and her partner's employment was as a cleaner. They had had no previous experience of speech and language therapy.

Dorothy

Dorothy's son had originally been allocated to the immediate therapy group but they failed to attend a number of appointments with the speech and language therapist over the course of the 12 months. At the end of the their involvement in the project, the child was four years, one month. He was still experiencing speech and language delay, which made him very difficult to understand. The mother felt that the child still needed to improve a great deal, but did not think that speech and language therapy had done very much for the child's problems. The family was made up of the mother, three older brothers and the child. All the other children had learned to talk without problems, although one child had been seen for an assessment by the speech and language therapist when he was school-aged. The mother was not in employment outside the home.

Wendy

Wendy's son had been allocated to the delayed therapy group. At the end of their involvement in the project, the child was four years, five months. He was still experiencing some speech difficulties, which his mother was not concerned about. She did not take up the offer of intensive therapy for her son at the end of the project because she felt his difficulties would resolve by themselves. The family was made up of the mother, one elder brother and the child. The elder brother had experienced no difficulties with his speech and language development and the mother had had no previous contact with a speech and language therapist. The mother worked on a part-time basis, as a hospital administrator.

Kate and Andrew

This was the third interview where the child's father was present along with the mother. In this case, the father had not been involved in taking his son to speech and language therapy and only made occasional comments in the course of the interview. Their son had originally been allocated to the delayed therapy group. They had asked for him to start receiving therapy after waiting for six months. They had then failed all but one of their speech and language therapy appointments since they had opted to change. At the end of their involvement in the project, the child was four years of age. He was still experiencing speech and language delay, which made him very difficult to understand. The family was made up of the mother, an elder sister and the child. The child's sister had learned to talk without problems. There was no previous experience of speech and language therapy. The mother was not in employment outside the home and the father was a mechanic.

Monica

Monica's daughter had originally been allocated to the delayed therapy group. She asked for therapy to begin after a wait of six months. At the end of their involvement in the project, the child was four years, six months. Monica's daughter was being assessed by a number of professionals at the time because she was thought to have a specific language impairment. She was experiencing serious problems with her understanding of language and the way in which she was putting sentences together. This family was made up of the mother, father and the child. They had had no previous experience of speech and language therapy. The mother was not in employment outside the home and the father worked as a lorry driver.

Isabel

Isabel's daughter had originally been allocated to the delayed therapy group. She had requested that her daughter's therapy start after waiting for six months. At the end of their involvement in the project, her child was three years, eight months. She was still experiencing speech problems. Isabel was glad that she had asked for therapy to begin and felt that it had helped her daughter. The family was made up of the mother, father, one older sister, the child and one younger sister. The older sister had had no difficulties with learning to talk and the younger sister was a young baby at the time of the interview. The family had had no prior contact with a speech and language therapist. Both parents worked outside the home as teachers.

Further reading

The following list of books and papers may be useful for people who wish to read further on the topics of speech and language development, speech and language delays and speech and language therapy for pre-school children. The list is in no way an exhaustive one.

Bishop D, Mogford K (eds) (1988) Language Development in Exceptional Circumstances. Hove: Lawrence Erlbaum Associates.

Cooke J, Williams D (1985) Working with Children's Language. Bicester: Winslow Press.

Cooper J, Moodley M, Reynell J (1978) Helping Language Development. London: Edward Arnold.

Crystal D (1986) Listen to your Child: A Parent's Guide to Children's Language Development. Harmondsworth: Penguin.

Enderby P, Emerson J (1995) 'Children with speech and language disorders.' In Enderby P, Emerson J (eds) Does Speech and Language Therapy Work? London: Whurr Publishers.

Kleinman A (1988) The Illness Narratives. Harvard: Basic Books.

Law J (1992) The Early Identification of Language Impairment in Children. London: Chapman Hall.

Law J (1994) Before School: A Handbook of Approaches to Intervention with Preschool Language Impaired Children. London: AFASIC.

Law J (1997) 'Evaluating early intervention for language impaired children: a review of the literature.' European Journal of Disorders of Communication 32: 1-14.

Law J, Boyle J, Harris F, Harkness A, Nye C (1998) 'Screening for speech and language delay: a systematic review of the literature.' Health Technology Assessment 2(9).

Law J, Parkinson A, Tamhne R (2000) Communication Difficulties in Childhood. Abingdon: Radcliffe Medical Press.

Whitehurst GJ, Fischel JE (1994) 'Practitioner review: early developmental language delay: what, if anything, should the clinician do about it?' Journal of Child Psychology and Psychiatry 35(4): 613-48.

Yule W, Rutter M (eds) (1987) Language Development and Language Disorder. London: MacKeith Press.

List of useful addresses

Royal College of Speech and Language Therapists (RCSLT)

2 White Hart Yard
London SE1 1NX
Telephone: 020 7378 1200
Fax: 020 7403 7254
Email: postmaster@rcslt.org
Website: www.rcslt.org

This is the professional body for speech and language therapists in the UK. A registered charity, it provides services for members and the general public. It can provide information on communication difficulties and offers a range of materials and publications.

Association for All Speech Impaired Children (AFASIC)

50–52 Great Sutton Street
London EC1V 0DJ
Telephone: 020 7490 9410
Helpline: 0845 355 5577
Fax: 020 7251 2834
Email: info@afasic.org.uk
Website: www.afasic.org.uk

This charity represents children and young people who are unable to communicate effectively because of a speech and language impairment. It provides support and information to professionals, parents and young adults with speech and language impairments. It also provides a range of leaflets, books and videos concerned with children's speech and language difficulties.

The Communications Forum

Camelford House
87–89 Albert Embankment
London SE1 7TP
Telephone: 020 7582 9200
Fax: 020 7582 9606
Email: cf@communicationsforum.org.uk
Website: www.communicationsforum.org.uk

The Forum brings together organizations concerned with the needs of people with speech and language impairments. It does not provide services but supports plans to increase awareness of communication issues among the general public and statutory and voluntary organizations.

I CAN

I CAN Central Office
4 Dyer's Buildings
Holborn
London EC1N 2QP
Telephone: 0870 010 4066
Fax: 0870 010 4067
Website: www.ican.org.uk

I CAN specializes in helping children, aged three to 16, who have speech and language difficulties. It runs three schools and is developing a network of pre-school services to meet the needs of young children with speech and language difficulties. It provides training for professionals and offers a range of publications.

Association of Speech and Language Therapists in Independent Practice (ASLTIIP, WSS)

Coleheath Bottom
Speen
Princes Risborough
Bucks HP27 0SZ
Telephone: 01494 488306
Fax: 01494 488590
Helpline: 0870 241 3357
Website: www.asltip.co.uk

This association is the official advisory and representative body for speech and language therapists working in private practice and is affiliated to the Royal College of Speech and Language Therapists. It provides information to the public about the independent sector.

Index